Praise for
The Glucose Revolution

■

"Forget *Sugar Busters*. Forget *The Zone*. If you want the real scoop on how carbohydrates and sugar affect your body, read this book by the world's leading researchers on the subject. It's the authoritative, last word on choosing foods to control your blood sugar."
—JEAN CARPER, best-selling author of
Miracle Cures, Stop Aging Now! and *Food—Your Miracle Medicine*

"The concept of the glycemic index has been distorted and bastardized by popular writers and diet gurus. Here, at last, is a book that explains what we know about the glycemic index and its importance in designing a diet for optimum health. Carbohydrates are not all bad. Read the good news about pasta and even—believe it or not—sugar!"
—ANDREW WEIL, M.D., University of Arizona College of Medicine,
author of *Spontaneous Healing* and *8 Weeks to Optimum Health*

"*The Glucose Revolution* is nutrition science for the 21st century. Clearly written, it gives the scientific rationale for why all carbohydrates are not created equal. It is a practical guide for both professionals and patients. The food suggestions and recipes are exciting and tasty."
—RICHARD N. PODELL, M.D., M.P.H.,
Clinical Professor, Department of Family Medicine,
UMDNJ–Robert Wood Johnson Medical School,
and co-author of *The G-Index Diet*: *The Missing Link That Makes
Permanent Weight Loss Possible*

"We've searched bookstores a long time for a clearly written book leading the way toward a healthier diet—high in whole, unprocessed complex carbohydrates and low in fat and refined foods. *The Glucose Revolution* is that book. It will transport you along a gentle, steady stream of information onto a sea of knowledge. If you want to see your diabetes and your kitchen in a whole new light, definitely get this book!"
—JOHN WALSH, P.A., C.D.E., and Ruth Roberts, M.A.,
authors of *Pumping Insulin* and *STOP the Rollercoaster*
and directors, The Diabetes Mall (www.diabetesnet.com)

■ ■ ■

"Mounting evidence indicates that refined carbohydrates and high glycemic index foods are contributing to the escalating epidemics of obesity and type 2 diabetes worldwide. This dietary pattern also appears to increase the risk of heart disease and stroke. The skyrocketing proportion of calories from added sugars and refined carbohydrates in westernized diets portends a future acceleration of these trends. *The Glucose Revolution* challenges traditional doctrines about optimal nutrition and the role of carbohydrates in health and disease. Brand-Miller and colleagues are to be congratulated for an eminently lucid and important book that explains the science behind the glycemic index and provides tools and strategies for modifying diet to incorporate this knowledge. I strongly recommend the book to both health professionals and the general public who could use this state-of-the-art information to improve health and well-being."

—JoAnn E. Manson, M.D., Dr.P.H.,
Professor of Medicine, Harvard Medical School and
Co-Director of Women's Health, Division of Preventive Medicine,
Brigham and Women's Hospital

"For decades we've known that success in athletics is based not only on how athletes train, but also on what they eat. Now *The Glucose Revolution* provides scientifically based nutritional advice to help athletes achieve peak performance and answers their many questions about what and when to eat before, during, and after competition. It clearly explains that eating high-carbohydrate foods when in training is not enough—the glycemic index must also be considered."

—Joe Friel, author of *The Triathlete's Training Bible*
and *The Cyclist's Training Bible*

"Here is at last a book explaining the importance of taking into consideration the glycemic index of foods for overall health, athletic performance, and in reducing the risk of heart disease and diabetes. The book clearly explains that there are different kinds of carbohydrates that work in different ways and why a universal recommendation to 'increase the carbohydrate content of your diet' is plainly simple and scientifically inaccurate. Everyone should put the glycemic index approach into practice."

—Artemis P. Simopoulos, M.D., senior author of
The Omega Diet and *The Healing Diet* and President,
The Center for Genetics, Nutrition and Health, Washington, D.C.

The
GLUCOSE REVOLUTION

The GLUCOSE Revolution

THE AUTHORITATIVE GUIDE TO
THE GLYCEMIC INDEX
THE GROUNDBREAKING MEDICAL DISCOVERY

JENNIE BRAND-MILLER, PH.D.

THOMAS M.S. WOLEVER, M.D., PH.D.

STEPHEN COLAGIURI, M.D.

KAYE FOSTER-POWELL, M. NUTR. & DIET.

ADAPTED BY JOHANNA BURANI, M.S., R.D., C.D.E.

■

MARLOWE & COMPANY
NEW YORK

Published by
Marlowe & Company
841 Broadway, 4th Floor
New York, NY 10003

This book is not intended to replace the services of a physician or dietitian.
Any application of the recommendations set forth in the following pages is at the
reader's discretion. The reader should consult with his or her own physician or dietitian
concerning the recommendations in this book.

First published in Australia in 1996 and 1998 under the title
The G.I. Factor by Hodder Headline Australia Pty Limited.

This edition is published by arrangement with
Hodder Headline Australia Pty Limited.

Library of Congress Cataloging-in-Publication Data

The glucose revolution: the authoritative guide to the glycemic index, the ground-
breaking medical discovery / by Jennie Brand Miller . . . [et al.].
p. cm.
Rev. ed. of: The G.I. factor / Jennie Brand Miller . . . [et al.].
Rydalmere, N.S.W.: Hodder Headline, 1998.
Includes bibliographical references and index.
ISBN 1-56924-660-2
1. Glycemic index. 2. Carbohydrates—Metabolism. 3. High-
carbohydrate diet. I. Miller, Jennie Brand. G.I. factor.
II. Miller, Jennie Brand.
Q701.G57 1999   98-56156
S12.3'96—dc21   CIP

First edition

Designed by Pauline Neuwirth, Neuwirth & Associates, Inc.
Distributed by Publishers Group West
Manufactured in the United States of America

CONTENTS

INTRODUCTION

The right kind of carbohydrate can make an important contribution to the quality of your life. *The Glucose Revolution* is
about the glycemic index (which we sometimes abbreviate as
G.I.). It will help you choose the right amount of carbohydrate and
the right sort of carbohydrate for your lifestyle and well-being. And
it will reduce your risk of developing heart disease or diabetes.

The glycemic index is a scientifically validated tool in the dietary
management of diabetes, weight loss, and athletic performance.
Foods with a **low glycemic index** help people control their hunger,
their appetite and their blood sugar levels. These foods actually help
athletes prolong endurance when eaten before an event. After the
first event, foods with a **high glycemic index** have been shown to
replenish energy stores faster and give athletes greater staying power
when competing in further events.

The glycemic index of foods is simply a ranking of foods based on their
immediate effect on blood glucose—or blood sugar levels.

- Carbohydrate foods that break down quickly during digestion have the
  highest glycemic indexes. Their blood sugar response is fast and high.
- Carbohydrates that break down slowly, releasing glucose gradually into
  the blood stream, have low glycemic index values.

THE GOOD NEWS

Our research on the glycemic index began in the late 1970s when
health authorities all over the world began to stress the importance

of high carbohydrate diets. Until then dietary fat had grabbed all the media attention (and to some extent this is still true). But low fat diets are by their very nature high in carbohydrate. The questions therefore became: *Which type of carbohydrate:*

- is best for overall health?
- can reduce our risk of diseases like heart disease or diabetes?
- is best for weight control?
- can optimize sports performance?

Our research since then has contributed to the worldwide recognition that the rate of carbohydrate digestion in the gastrointestinal (digestive) tract has important implications for everybody.

Although the glycemic index has been well described in scientific journals and nutrition text books over the past decade, it has been controversial, particularly in the United States. At present the American Diabetes Association (ADA) does not endorse the use of the glycemic index in the dietary management of diabetes, although other diabetes associations around the world do, including the Canadian Diabetes Association, the European Association for the Study of Diabetes, Diabetes Australia, and the International Diabetes Institute. The ADA believes that differences in the glycemic index among foods are not large enough to warrant changes to the diet, especially in the context of mixed, or real meals. However, a steady stream of studies in the last few years has convinced many people in the United States, as elsewhere, of the usefulness of the glycemic index. Additionally, efforts by food manufacturers to produce foods with low glycemic index values may also help broaden the public's interest in and acceptance of the glycemic index.

Meanwhile, we believe that it is time to spread the good news to a wider audience and to broadcast the fact that there are different types of carbohydrate that work in different ways. So, we wrote *The Glucose Revolution* to give you a guide to the physiological effects of foods on your blood sugar levels. Why do we call it the *glucose revolution*? Because the news we present about foods—and especially carbohydrates—is truly revolutionary. It will change the way you think about the foods—especially the carbohydrates—you eat.

The good news is that the glycemic index provides an easier and more effective way to win the battle of the bulge and control fluctuations in blood sugar (glucose). People with diabetes or heart disease in the family, as well as serious athletes will welcome the news. For some people it will lift the great burden of guilt about eating.

BLOOD SUGAR OR BLOOD GLUCOSE?

Blood sugar and blood glucose mean the same thing, although the latter is technically more correct. However, we use the term blood sugar in this book because it is more widely understood. "Glycemic" (pronounced gly-semic) refers to "blood sugar."

In this edition of the book we give you all the details on the glycemic index plus recipes, meal plans and the very latest findings including:

- The benefit of vinegar and lemon juice on G.I.
- Recent studies from Harvard University
- Glycemic index figures for recently tested foods.

KEY POINTS ABOUT THE GLYCEMIC INDEX

- The modern diet is too high in saturated fat and fast-release carbohydrates.

- The carbohydrate we eat is digested and absorbed too quickly because most modern starchy foods have a high glycemic index.

- The glycemic index is a ranking of foods based on their overall effect on blood sugar levels (low G.I. means a smaller rise of blood sugar).

- Middle-aged people who follow a low G.I. diet may be less likely to develop diabetes and heart disease.

- Low G.I. diets can help control established diabetes.

- Low G.I. diets can help people lose weight.

- Low G.I. diets may help lower blood lipids.

- Low G.I. diets can improve the body's sensitivity to insulin.

- Low G.I. foods reduce the glycemic index of the meal as a whole.

- A high glycemic index food + a low glycemic index food = an intermediate glycemic index meal.

- To make the change to a low G.I. diet use more:

  - low G.I. breakfast cereals (based on wheat bran, psyllium, barley and oats)
  - "Grainy" breads made with whole seeds of barley, rye, oats, soy and wheat
  - pasta and rice in place of potatoes
  - vinegar and lemon juice dressings

DISPELLING SOME MYTHS ABOUT FOOD

This book dispels many myths about food and carbohydrate. We now know from our scientific research into the glycemic index that the following popular beliefs about food and carbohydrate are not true.

MYTH 1   Sugar is fattening.
Not true. Sugar has no special fattening properties. It is no more likely to be turned into fat than any other carbohydrate. Sugar, which is often present in foods high in energy and fat, may sometimes seem to be "turned to fat," but it's the total energy (calories) rather than the sugar in those energy-dense foods that may contribute to new stores of body fat.

MYTH 2   **Sugar is the worst thing for people with diabetes.**
          Not true. Sugar and sugary foods in normal servings have
          no greater effect on blood sugar levels than many starchy
          foods. Saturated fat is far worse for people with diabetes.

MYTH 3   **Sugar causes diabetes.**
          Not true. Sugar has no unique role in causing diabetes.
          Foods that produce high blood sugar levels may increase
          the risk of diabetes, but sugar has only a moderate effect.

MYTH 4   **All starches are slowly digested in the intestine.**
          Not true. Some starch, like that in potatoes, is digested
          in a flash, causing a greater rise in blood sugar than
          many sugar-containing foods.

MYTH 5   **Hunger pangs are inevitable if you want to lose weight.**
          Not true. High carbohydrate foods, especially those with
          a low glycemic index (e.g. rolled oats and pasta), will
          sustain the feeling of fullness almost to the next meal.

MYTH 6   **Starchy foods like bread and potatoes are fattening.**
          Not true. Bread and potatoes are rich in carbohydrate—
          the easiest fuel for our bodies to burn—and therefore
          among the best foods you can eat to help you lose weight.

MYTH 7   **Starches are best for optimum athletic performance.**
          Not true. In many instances starchy foods (e.g. potatoes)
          are too bulky to eat in the quantities needed for active
          athletes.

MYTH 8   **Foods high in fat are more filling.**
          Not true. Recent studies show that high fat foods are
          among the least filling. It is extremely easy to "passively
          overconsume" foods like potato chips and french fries.

MYTH 9   **Diets high in sugar are less nutritious.**
          Not true. Studies have shown that diets high in sugar

(from a range of sources including dairy products and fruit) often have higher levels of micronutrients such as calcium, riboflavin and vitamin C than low sugar diets.

MYTH 10 Sugar goes hand in hand with dietary fat.
Not true. The reality is that diets high in sugar are usually low in fat and vice versa. Most sources of fat in the diet are not sweetened (e.g. potato chips) and most sources of sugar contain no fat (e.g. soft drinks). Yes, there are many foods high in both fat and sugar (chocolate, ice cream, cakes, cookies) but these usually represent less than 10 percent of energy intake.

WHO IS THIS BOOK FOR?

The Glucose Revolution is for just about everybody. In particular it is for people who will gain most from putting the glycemic index approach into practice—people who have or are at risk for diabetes or heart disease, people who are overweight as well as athletes. Most people have some notion of how blood sugar rises and falls. However, much of the information currently in print about food and blood sugar is wrong. *The Glucose Revolution* gives you the true story about carbohydrate and the blood glucose—or blood sugar—connection.

This book will give people with diabetes a new lease on life, literally! Many people with diabetes find that despite doing all the right things, their blood sugar levels remain too high. The glycemic index allows people with diabetes to choose the right kind of carbohydrate for blood sugar control.

This book gives athletes the competitive edge over their rivals by allowing them to choose the best carbohydrate for optimum sports performance. Some athletes already know something about carbohydrate loading but think that it sounds too complicated. Others are now following a high carbohydrate diet but wonder whether some types of carbohydrate are better than others.

The Glucose Revolution also helps answer the questions about sugar from worried parents who are generally concerned about their family's health and well-being.

THIS BOOK WILL GIVE

PEOPLE WITH DIABETES

A NEW LEASE ON LIFE, LITERALLY!

HOW YOU CAN USE THIS BOOK

Please don't be tempted to skip the early chapters of this book and jump straight into the specific applications of the glycemic index for weight loss, diabetes, heart disease, or athletic performance. We recommend you read the introductory chapters as they will give you a complete overview of the carbohydrate story. The facts we reveal about carbohydrate will surprise many people—facts that can make life a lot easier.

Part I contains the most up-to-date information about what makes a balanced diet and why—information based on scientific research, clinical trials and real-life experiences. It stresses the value of a low G.I. and low fat diet for everybody. It tells you which types of carbohydrate are best and why. It explains why the glycemic index is the best tool for choosing the right types of carbohydrate for your needs and your lifestyle. Separate chapters cover how you can use the glycemic index to lose weight, lower blood sugar levels, reduce blood fats and improve athletic performance.

In Part II we show you how you can include more of the right sort of carbohydrate in your diet, give hints for meal preparation, and practical tips and food combinations to help you to make the glycemic index work for you throughout the day. This section includes over fifty imaginative and delicious recipes for breakfast, lunch, dinner and in-between snacks which we have developed and tested along with their glycemic index and nutritional analysis.

If it's just the glycemic index values you are after, you'll find them in Part III, which contains an A to Z listing of foods, their fat and carbohydrate content, and their glycemic index values. This is the largest complete list of glycemic index values for different foods ever published in a book.

Finally there's a complete list of scientific references on pages 255 to 262 to back up everything we say.

Part 1

WHAT YOU NEED TO KNOW ABOUT THE GLYCEMIC INDEX

■

Chapter 1

WHAT'S WRONG WITH TODAY'S DIET?

WHAT OUR ANCESTORS ATE

For the past 10,000 years, our ancestors survived on a high carbohydrate and low fat diet. They ate their carbohydrate in the form of beans, vegetables and whole cereal grains. They ate their sugars in fibrous fruits and berries. Food preparation was a simple process: grinding food between stones and cooking it over the heat of an open fire. The result of this process was that all food was digested and absorbed slowly and the usual blood sugar rise was gradual and prolonged.

This diet was ideal as far as their bodies were concerned because it provided slow-release energy that helped to delay hunger pangs and provided fuel for working muscles long after the meal was eaten. It was also kind to the pancreas.

As time passed, flours were ground more and more finely and bran was separated completely from the white flour. With the advent of high speed roller mills in the nineteenth century, it was possible to produce white flour so fine that it resembled talcum powder in appearance and texture. These fine white flours have always been highly prized because they make soft bread and light, airy sponge cakes. As incomes grew, the peas and beans that were staples of the diet were cast aside and meat consumption increased. As a consequence, the composition of the average diet changed: we began to eat more fat and the type of carbohydrate in our diet changed, becoming more quickly digested and absorbed. Something we didn't expect happened, too. The blood sugar rise after a meal was higher and more prolonged, stimulating the pancreas to produce more insulin (see box).

THE PANCREAS PRODUCES INSULIN

The pancreas is a vital organ near the stomach. Its main job is to produce the hormone insulin. Carbohydrate stimulates the secretion of insulin more than any other component of food. The slow absorption of the carbohydrate in our food means that the pancreas doesn't have to work so hard and produces less insulin. If the pancreas is over-stimulated over a long period of time, it may become "exhausted" and type 2 diabetes develops in genetically susceptible individuals. Even without diabetes, high insulin levels are undesirable because they increase the risk of heart disease.

So not only did we have higher blood sugar levels after a meal, we had higher insulin responses as well. Insulin is a hormone that is needed for carbohydrate metabolism, but it has a profound effect on the development of many diseases. Medical experts now believe that high insulin levels are one of the key factors responsible for heart disease and hypertension. Insulin influences the way we metabolize foods, determining whether we burn fat or carbohydrate to meet our energy needs and ultimately determining whether we store fat in our body.

Thus one of the most important ways in which our diet differs from that of our ancestors is the speed of carbohydrate digestion and the resulting effect on blood sugar and insulin levels. In summary, traditional diets all around the world contained slowly digested and absorbed carbohydrate—foods that we now know have a low glycemic index. In contrast, modern diets with their quickly digested fine white flours are based on foods with a high glycemic index.

WHAT WE REALLY NEED TO EAT
FOR HEALTH AND GROWTH

Food is part of our culture and way of life. Our food choices are determined by many factors ranging from religious beliefs to the deliciously sensual role that food plays in our lives. For babies, food has a comforting role to play, beyond meeting the immediate physical need. For adults, food reflects status—we prepare special meals for special occasions and for special guests to show respect or friendship.

It is no wonder that with so many factors influencing our food choices, we tend to overlook the very basic role food plays in the nourishment and growth of our bodies. In a busy lifestyle, it's easy to see food simply as a solution to overcoming hunger. In other circumstances we focus on the social aspects of food and eat too much.

In 1992, the United States Department of Agriculture (USDA) developed the Food Guide Pyramid, a food model which guides us on the types and amounts of foods we should be eating daily for health. For many reasons our eating habits today fall very short of these recommendations.

Calorie-laden foods (sometimes called energy dense foods), such as alcohol, chocolate, potato chips and candy, provide few nutrients for a lot of calories. For this reason they are referred to as "indulgences" and are best limited to no more than one to two servings per day.

WHAT'S WRONG WITH TODAY'S DIET?

Today's Western diet is the product of industrialization based on inventions ranging from Jethro Tull's seed drill (in 1701) to the high speed steel roller mills for milling cereals (in the nineteenth century) and advances in processing food to give it a longer shelf life. The

FOOD GUIDE PYRAMID
A GUIDE TO DAILY FOOD CHOICES

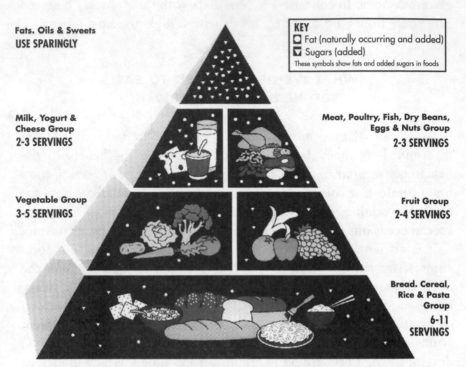

Source: United States Department of Agriculture and United States Department of Health and Human Services

benefits are many. We have a plentiful, relatively cheap, palatable (some would say too palatable) and safe food supply. Gone are the days of monotonous fare, gaps in the food supply, weevil-infested and adulterated food. Long gone are widespread vitamin deficiencies such as scurvy and pellagra. Today's food manufacturers work hard to bring us irresistible products that meet the demands of both gourmets and health conscious consumers.

Many of the new foods are still based on our staple cereals—wheat, corn, and oats—but the original grain has been ground down to produce fine flours with small particle size that produces the best quality breads, cakes, cookies, breakfast cereals, and snack foods.

Cereal chemists and bakers know that the finest particle size flour produces the most palatable and shelf-stable end product. But this striving for excellence in one area has resulted in unforeseen problems in another. Today's staple carbohydrate foods, including ordinary bread, are quickly digested and absorbed. The resulting effect on blood sugar levels has created a problem for many of us.

WITH A WAVE OF THE FAT WAND . . .

The other undesirable aspect of the modern diet is its high fat content. Food manufacturers, bakers and chefs know we love to eat fat. We love its creaminess and mouth feel and find it easy to consume in excess. It makes our meat more tender, our vegetables and salads more palatable and our sweet foods even more desirable. We prefer potatoes as French fries or potato chips, to have our fish battered and fried, and our pastas in rich creamy sauces. With a wave of the fat wand, bland high carbohydrate foods like rice and oats are magically transformed into very palatable, calorie-laden foods such as fried rice and sweetened granola. In fact, when you analyze it, much of our diet today is an undesirable but delicious combination of both fat and quickly digested carbohydrate.

WHAT'S WRONG WITH OUR WAY OF EATING?

- The modern diet is too high in saturated fat and too high in quick-release carbohydrate.
- The carbohydrate we eat is digested and absorbed too quickly because most modern starchy foods have a high glycemic index.

WHY WE NEED TO EAT MORE CARBOHYDRATE

For once the experts on health are nearly unanimous. Most agree that the food we eat for breakfast, lunch and dinner and for those in-between snacks should be low in fat and high in carbohydrate. The same diet that helps prevent our becoming overweight also reduces our risk of developing heart disease, diabetes and many types of cancer. This same high carbohydrate and low fat diet improves athletic performance.

But the story doesn't finish there. To reduce the fat content of our diet, we need to eat carbohydrate more. Carbohydrate should be the main source of calories in our food, not fat. Carbohydrate and fat have a reciprocal relationship in our diet. If we eat more high carbohydrate foods, they tend to displace the high fat foods from our diet. The new emphasis on eating lots of high carbohydrate foods has focused attention on the differences among carbohydrates.

SO, WHAT IS A BALANCED DIET?

It makes sense to balance our food intake with the rate our bodies use it. This way, we maintain a steady weight. These days, however, this balance is difficult to achieve. It is very easy to overeat. Refined foods, convenience foods and fast foods frequently lack fiber and conceal fat so that before we feel full, we have overdosed on calories. It is even easier not to exercise. It takes longer to walk somewhere than it does to drive (except perhaps in rush hour). With intake exceeding output on a regular basis, the result for too many of us is gaining weight.

We need to adapt our lifestyle to our high caloric diet and fewer physical demands. It's become very important to catch bursts of physical activity wherever we can to increase our energy output. It may mean using the stairs instead of the elevator, taking a 10 minute walk at lunch time, jogging on a treadmill while you watch the news, reading on the stationary bike, making more effort in the garden, walking to the store to get the Sunday paper, parking a half a mile from work, or taking the dog for a walk each night. Whatever it means, do it. Even housework burns calories. All these seemingly small bursts of activity accumulate to increase our calorie output. You don't have to take exercise seriously, just do it regularly.

While you work on increasing your energy output, the glycemic index can help you select the best foods to balance your intake. Its high carbohydrate basis ensures a filling diet which isn't packed with calories.

So, our first message is to reduce the amount of fat you eat. This applies to all sorts of fat: saturated, polyunsaturated, monounsaturated. (Caution: A low fat diet is good for most of us, but it is not appropriate for children who rely on fat for growth.) But the flip side of this message is to eat more carbohydrate because this can help reduce your fat intake. The following chapters tell you how you can eat more carbohydrate and which foods you should choose to replace fatty foods. It also goes one step further and tells you which carbohydrates are best for health—and why.

Chapter 2

THE HIGH CARBOHYDRATE DIET

HOW DOES CARBOHYDRATE WORK?

SO, WHAT MAKES A HIGH CARBOHYDRATE DIET?

HOW MUCH CARBOHYDRATE DO YOU NEED IN A DAY?

CARBOHYDRATE REQUIREMENTS FOR SMALL EATERS

CARBOHYDRATE REQUIREMENTS FOR AVERAGE EATERS

CARBOHYDRATE REQUIREMENTS FOR BIG EATERS

WHAT'S WRONG WITH THIS MENU?

WHAT ABOUT THE DIFFERENT TYPES OF CARBOHYDRATE?

THE CARBOHYDRATE—GLYCEMIC INDEX LINK

Our bodies burn fuel all the time and the fuel our bodies like best is carbohydrate. Just as you would never try to run your car without gasoline—its essential energy source—you should not try to run your body without carbohydrate—your body's preferred energy source. Carbohydrate is the main fuel we use when we walk, talk, think, move, scratch, sneeze, jump, or sleep. Everything!

You might think of carbohydrate as the all important ingredient that makes foods taste sweet. It is also the starchy part of foods like rice, bread, potatoes and pasta. In fact, carbohydrate is the most widely consumed nutrient in the world, after water. It's important to the human body because it yields glucose. Glucose is so important that if your diet doesn't provide enough carbohydrate, your brain signals a shortage of glucose, and muscle tissue will be broken down to supply the shortfall. This basically means that you lose body muscle to feed your brain. Carbohydrate also displaces fat from the diet. While not all fats are bad (monounsaturated and polyunsaturated are fine), they are all easy to overconsume, i.e., eat in excess of your requirements. It's easy to put on excess weight if your diet is dominated by fats. Ideally, 50 to 60 percent of your daily calorie intake should come from carbohydrate.

HOW DOES CARBOHYDRATE WORK?

The usual sources of glucose for the body are the sugars and starches in food. To make use of these, the body must first break them down in the gut into a form that can be absorbed and which the cells can use. This process is called digestion.

Digestion starts in the mouth when **amylase**, the digestive enzyme in saliva, is incorporated into the food by chewing. The activity of this enzyme stops in the stomach. Most of the digestion continues only when the carbohydrate reaches the small intestine. In the small intestine, amylase from pancreatic juice breaks down the large molecules of starch into short chain molecules. These and any **disaccharide** sugars are then broken into simpler monosaccharides by enzymes in the wall of the intestine. The **monosaccharides** that result, **glucose, fructose** and **galactose**, are absorbed from the small intestine into the blood stream where they are available as a source of energy to the cells.

The body maintains a certain level of glucose in the blood to serve the brain and central nervous system. To ensure a readily available supply of glucose, the body stores glucose in the muscles and the liver. This stored glucose is called glycogen. If you are eating insufficient carbohydrate, these glycogen stores will be broken down and converted to glucose. Once the body has used up its glycogen it will start breaking down muscle protein to synthesize glucose for the vital organs. A low carbohydrate diet will make you feel headachy and unwell and causes loss of lean muscle tissue and water—two things you need to hang on to! It will not help you lose weight because the body's fat stores cannot be converted to glucose.

WHAT IS CARBOHYDRATE?

Carbohydrate is a part of food. Starch is a carbohydrate, so too are sugars and certain types of fiber. Starches are nature's reserves created by energy from the sun, carbon dioxide and water. The building block of starch is glucose, a single sugar.

The simplest form of carbohydrate is a single sugar molecule. Chemically, this sugar molecule is known as a **monosaccharide** (**mono** meaning one, **saccharide** meaning sweet). Glucose is a single sugar molecule which occurs in foods and is the most common source of fuel for the cells of the human body.

If two sugar molecules are joined together, the result is a **disaccharide** (**di** meaning two). Sucrose, or common table sugar, is a disaccharide.

Starches are long chains of sugar molecules joined together like the beads in a string of pearls. They are called **polysaccharides** (**poly** meaning many). Starches are not sweet tasting.

Dietary fibers also have a complex structure, containing many different sorts of sugar molecules. They are different from starches and sugars in that they are not broken down by human digestive enzymes. Fiber reaches the large intestine without change. Once there, bacteria begin to ferment and break down the fibers.

SUGARS FOUND IN FOOD

Monosaccharides
(single sugar molecules)

Disaccharides
(two single sugar molecules joined together)

glucose
fructose
galactose

maltose = glucose + glucose
sucrose = glucose + fructose
lactose = glucose + galactose

■ ■ ■

SOURCES OF CARBOHYDRATE

Carbohydrate mainly comes from plant foods, such as cereal grains, fruits, vegetables and legumes (peas and beans). Milk products also contain carbohydrate. Some foods contain a large amount of carbohydrate (e.g. cereals, potatoes, legumes) while other foods are very dilute sources (e.g. carrots, broccoli, salad vegetables). The dilute sources can be eaten freely, but they won't provide anywhere near enough carbohydrate for our high-carbohydrate diet. A salad is not a meal and must be complemented by a carbohydrate-dense food such as bread. The following list includes foods that are high in carbohydrate and provide very little fat. Eat lots of them, sparing the butter, margarine and oil during their preparation.

Cereal grains including rice, wheat, oats, barley, rye and anything made from them (bread, pasta, breakfast cereal, flour).

Fruits such as apples, oranges, bananas, grapes, peaches, melons etc.

Vegetables such as potatoes, yams, sweet corn, taro and sweet potato are all high in carbohydrate.

Legumes, peas and beans including baked beans, lentils, kidney beans, chickpeas etc.

Milk contains carbohydrate, in the form of milk sugar or lactose. Lactose is the first carbohydrate we encounter as infants. Use low fat or skim milk and yogurt to minimize fat intake.

TOP 20 SOURCES OF CARBOHYDRATE IN THE AMERICAN DIET*

1. Potatoes (mashed or baked)	8. Pizza	16. Table sugar
2. White bread	9. Pasta	17. Jam
3. Cold breakfast cereal	10. Muffins	18. Cranberry juice
4. Dark bread	11. Fruit punch	19. French fries
5. Orange juice	12. Coca-Cola	20. Candy
6. Banana	13. Apple	
7. White rice	14. Skim milk	
	15. Pancake	

Source: Dr. Simin Liu, Harvard University School of Public Health.

*This data represents the findings of the Harvard Nurses' Health Study.

SO, WHAT MAKES A HIGH CARBOHYDRATE DIET?

Eating a high carbohydrate diet means:

- eating carbohydrate-rich foods at every meal and making sure that carbohydrates form a large proportion of the meal,
- eating carbohydrate-rich foods for snacks,
- including at least the minimum quantity of carbohydrate foods suggested for small eaters (see page 16).

Eating a high carbohydrate diet also means:

- not eating too much fat. High fat foods are a concentrated source of calories. It takes only a small extra amount of them to throw your diet out of balance. Monounsaturated and polyunsaturated fats may have desirable effects on blood lipid levels but *all* fats have the same energy value and same propensity for "overconsumption."

HOW MUCH CARBOHYDRATE DO YOU NEED IN A DAY?

Most of the world's peoples eat a high carbohydrate diet based on staples such as rice, corn, millet and wheat-based foods like pasta or bread. In developing countries, carbohydrate may form 70 to 80 percent of a person's calorie intake. In developed countries the intake may be half this. In the United States and Canada, the United Kingdom, Australia and New Zealand, carbohydrate typically contributes only 40 to 45 percent of calorie intake. In these countries, carbohydrate, the body's vital energy source, tends to be crowded out by fat.

Current recommendations suggest that we take at least 50 to 60 percent of our total calories as carbohydrate. To do this we need to consume 150 grams of carbohydrate for every 1000 calories. For a low calorie diet (1200 calories) it means eating about 175 grams of carbohydrate per day (equivalent to about 12 slices of bread). A young, active person with higher energy requirements, say in the order of 2000 calories, would require 300 grams of carbohydrate (equivalent to about 20 slices of bread). As an example of what this looks like we have calculated a sample carbohydrate intake for small eaters and bigger eaters (see pages 16 to 18).

The number of calories and hence the amount of carbohydrate needed varies greatly between people. Your energy requirements depend on your age, sex, activity level and body size. It is not possible to publish standard figures that will apply to every reader. If you want more information on your own specific calorie and carbohydrate needs, we suggest that you consult a dietitian. Dietitians can help you assess your calorie requirements and calculate exactly how much carbohydrate you need. Most of us don't need to keep count of the number of grams of carbohydrate we eat every day. But for some people, like athletes, it may be necessary to keep a watch to make sure that they are eating enough carbohydrate.

HOW TO FIND A DIETITIAN

If you want to consult a dietitian about your calorie requirements and how much carbohydrate you need, look in the Yellow Pages under Dietitians, or call the American Dietetic Association's Consumer Nutrition Hotline (800-366-1655) or go to ADA's home page: http://www.eatright.org/. Make sure that the person you choose has the letters R.D. (Registered Dietitian) after his or her name.

However, if you are looking at ways to improve your own diet there are two important things to remember:

1. Identify the sources of fat and look at ways you can reduce it. Don't go overboard—the body needs **some** fat in the diet.
2. Check whether you need to add more carbohydrate to your diet and eat more. Most people don't eat enough.

Note: A low fat diet is not appropriate for children under five years of age. They need the extra energy provided by fat for normal growth and development.

CARBOHYDRATE REQUIREMENTS FOR SMALL EATERS

You might consider yourself a small eater if you:
- are a small-framed female,
- have a small appetite,
- do very little physical activity,
- are trying to lose weight.

Even the smallest eater needs the following carbohydrate foods every day:

- around 4 slices of bread or the equivalent (crackers, rolls, English muffins) PLUS
- at least 3 pieces of fruit or the equivalent (juice, dried fruit) PLUS
- about 1 cup of high carbohydrate cooked vegetables (corn, legumes, potato, sweet potato) PLUS
- about 1½ cups of cereal or grain food (breakfast cereal, cooked rice or pasta, or other grains) PLUS
- at least 1½ cups of fat free or 1% milk or yogurt. This includes milk in your tea and coffee and with your cereal.

If this amount of food sounds right for you, try it as a minimum amount of carbohydrate. This supplies 200 grams of carbohydrate, suitable for a 1500 calorie diet. Listen to your appetite if it demands more.

HOW COULD YOU CHANGE YOUR DIET?

Some of the most common changes that people tell us they have made to their diet using the glycemic index are:
- Eating whole grain breads.
- Eating more fruit and yogurt.
- Eating lots of pasta, beans and vegetables.

■ ■ ■

CARBOHYDRATE REQUIREMENTS FOR AVERAGE EATERS

The picture of an average eater would fit you if you are:

- doing regular physical activity (but not strenuous exercise),
- an adult of average frame size.

Average eaters need to eat:

- around 6 slices of bread or the equivalent (crackers, rolls, English muffins) PLUS
- about 4 pieces of fruit or the equivalent (juice, dried fruit) PLUS
- 1 cup of high carbohydrate vegetables (corn, legumes, potato, sweet potato) PLUS
- at least 2 cups of cereal or grain food (breakfast cereal or cooked rice, or pasta or other grain) PLUS
- 2 cups of fat free or 1% milk or yogurt.

This provides 264 grams of carbohydrate which is suitable for a 2000 calorie diet. This is appropriate for a young, active adult of average build.

Carbohydrate is the most satiating of all nutrients. This simply means that it satisfies your appetite and fills you up. Overconsumption of food is highly unlikely on a high carbohydrate and low fat diet. So, base your diet on high fiber carbohydrate foods like whole grain breads, cereals, fruit, vegetables and legumes and let your appetite dictate how much you need to eat.

CARBOHYDRATE REQUIREMENTS FOR BIG EATERS

Typical big eaters are:

- teenagers and young adults,
- people working as laborers,
- people doing regular strenuous exercise.

Big eaters need to eat:

- at least 8 slices of bread or the equivalent (crackers, rolls, English muffins) PLUS
- 4 pieces of fruit or the equivalent (juice, dried fruit) PLUS
- at least 2 cups of high carbohydrate vegetables (corn, legumes, potato, sweet potato) PLUS
- at least 2 cups of cereal or grain food (breakfast cereal or cooked rice, or pasta or other grain) PLUS
- 2½ cups of fat free or 1% milk or the equivalent (yogurt, ice cream)

This provides 330 grams of carbohydrate which is suitable for a 2500 calorie diet.

An athlete who is training hard would generally need to eat double this quantity of carbohydrate.

WHAT'S WRONG WITH THIS MENU?

Take a look at this menu. To many people, it may sound very familiar.

- **Breakfast**
  2 slices whole wheat toast with butter and jam
  coffee with cream, no sugar

- **Mid-morning Snack**
  an apple
  tea or decaffeinated coffee with milk

- **Lunch**
  a large mixed salad containing a variety of vegetables with a slice of cheddar cheese, an egg, plus a few crackers (no butter)
  coffee with cream, no sugar

■ ■ ■

- **Dinner**
  grilled beef rib-steak
  carrots, beans, cauliflower and 1 potato
  coffee with cream, no sugar

- **Late Snack**
  a handful of peanuts
Total energy: 1400 calories
Fat: 75 grams
Carbohydrate: 105 grams
Fiber: 20 grams

Looking at an analysis of this day we can see that:

1. **It is low in carbohydrate. Only 30 percent of the total calories
   are supplied by carbohydrate. It is widely recommended that at
   least 50 percent of our daily calories should come from carbohydrate.**

To improve this diet it is essential to add some carbohydrate.

- Include a bowl of cereal and a piece of fruit with breakfast.
- Change the crackers at lunch to 2 slices of whole grain bread.
- Substitute the peanuts with a low fat yogurt as the late night
  snack.
- Add an ear of corn to the evening vegetables.
- Try a piece of fresh fruit or some unsweetened canned peaches for
  dessert.

2. **It is high in fat. Forty-six percent of the total calories are provided by fat. It is widely recommended that less than 30 percent
   of calories should come from fat.**

To improve this diet, take away some fat.

- Halve the amount of butter used on toast, or replace with a small
  amount of jam.

- Use a slice of low fat cheese **or** ham **or** an egg for lunch, not cheese **and** egg.
- Cut down on the portion of meat—select a small piece of fillet instead.
- Give up the peanuts! Substitute low fat yogurt instead, or unsweetened canned fruit, or low fat ice cream with fruit salad.

To work out the percentage of calories supplied by carbohydrate, the grams of carbohydrate are multiplied by 4 (the number of calories supplied per gram of carbohydrate) and then divided by the total number of calories. Thus: $(105 \times 4 \times 100)/1500 = 28$ percent

---

WHAT ABOUT THE DIFFERENT TYPES OF CARBOHYDRATE?

Traditionally, carbohydrate has been classified in terms of its chemical structure. We now know from scientific research and clinical trials with real people that the whole concept of simple and complex carbohydrates does not tell us anything about how they will actually behave in the body. Until recently, it was widely believed that complex carbohydrates, or starches such as rice and potato, were slowly digested and absorbed and therefore caused only a small rise in blood sugar level. Simple sugars, on the other hand, were assumed to be digested and absorbed quickly, producing a large and rapid increase in blood sugar. These assumptions were wrong.

FORGET ABOUT THE WORDS

SIMPLE AND COMPLEX CARBOHYDRATE.

THINK IN TERMS OF

LOW GLYCEMIC INDEX AND HIGH GLYCEMIC INDEX.

THE CARBOHYDRATE—GLYCEMIC INDEX LINK

Newer studies are revealing that the physiological responses to food (how food acts in the body) are far more complex than was previously appreciated. What is true is that different carbohydrate-containing foods do have different effects on blood sugar levels.

Only in recent years have scientists begun to study the actual blood sugar responses to hundreds of different foods in healthy people as well as people with diabetes. They gave them real foods—not solutions of sugars and starches in water. They measured the blood sugar levels at frequent intervals, for as long as two to three hours after the meal. To compare foods according to their true physiological effect on blood sugar levels, they came up with the term "glycemic index."

The glycemic index is a ranking of foods from 0 to 100 that tells us whether a food will raise blood sugar levels dramatically, moderately, or just a little.

This research has turned some widely held beliefs upside down.

The first surprise was that many starchy foods (bread, potatoes and many types of rice) are digested and absorbed very quickly, not slowly, as had always been assumed.

Secondly, research has found that moderate amounts of most sugary foods (candy, ice cream etc.) did not produce dramatic rises in blood sugar as had always been thought. The truth was that foods containing sugar actually showed quite low-to-moderate blood sugar responses, lower than foods like bread.

So, it is time to forget the old distinctions that were made between starchy foods and sugary foods or simple versus complex carbohydrate. These distinctions are based on chemical analysis of the food, which does **not** reflect the effects of these foods in the body. The glycemic index takes us nearer to a full understanding of how the body responds to carbohydrate foods.

■ ■ ■

THE GLYCEMIC INDEX

IS A RANKING OF FOODS

BASED ON THEIR OVERALL EFFECTS

ON BLOOD SUGAR LEVELS.

The next chapter tells you all about the glycemic index.

Chapter 3

ALL ABOUT
THE GLYCEMIC INDEX

THE KEY IS THE RATE OF DIGESTION

WHY THE GLYCEMIC INDEX IS SO IMPORTANT

CAN THE GLYCEMIC INDEX BE APPLIED TO REAL MEALS?

WHAT GIVES ONE FOOD A HIGH GLYCEMIC INDEX
AND ANOTHER FOOD A LOW ONE?

HOW DOES THE GLYCEMIC INDEX RELATE TO
BLOOD INSULIN LEVELS?

THE EFFECT OF FAT AND PROTEIN
ON THE GLYCEMIC INDEX

WHAT EFFECT ON BLOOD SUGAR LEVELS DOES AN
INCREASED CARBOHYDRATE INTAKE HAVE?

THE EFFECT OF SUGAR ON THE GLYCEMIC INDEX

THE EFFECT OF FIBER ON THE GLYCEMIC INDEX

THE POWERFUL EFFECT OF ACID ON G.I.

CAN I MEASURE MY OWN
G.I. BLOOD SUGAR RESPONSE?

The glycemic index concept was first developed in 1981 by a team of scientists led by Dr. David Jenkins, a professor of nutrition at the University of Toronto, Canada, to help determine which foods were best for people with diabetes. At that time, the diet for people with diabetes was based on a system of carbohydrate exchanges or portions, which was complicated and not very logical. The carbohydrate exchange system assumed that all starchy foods produce the same effect on blood sugar levels even though some earlier studies had already proven this was not correct. Jenkins was one of the first researchers to question this assumption and to investigate how real foods behave in the bodies of real people.

Jenkins's approach attracted a great deal of attention because it was so logical and systematic. He and his colleagues had tested a large number of common foods. Some of their results were surprising. Ice cream, for example, despite its sugar content, had much less effect on blood sugar than ordinary bread. Over the next fifteen years medical researchers and scientists around the world, including the authors of this book, tested the effect of many foods on blood sugar levels and developed a new concept of classifying carbohydrates based on their glycemic index.

For some years the glycemic index was a very controversial area. There were avid proponents and opponents of this new approach to classifying carbohydrate. The two sides almost came to blows at conferences aimed at reaching a consensus.

Initially, there was some justifiable criticism. In the early days of research, there was no evidence that glycemic index values for single foods could be applied to real, or what are also called mixed meals, or that the approach brought long-term benefits. There were no studies of its reproducibility or the consistency of glycemic index values from one country to another. Many of the early studies used healthy volunteers, and there was no evidence that the results could be applied to people with diabetes. But now the evidence is in and we know that the glycemic index is a **valid** and **clinically proven** tool in its applications to diabetes, appetite control and athletics. To date, clinical studies in the United States, United Kingdom, France, Italy, Sweden, Australia and Canada all have proven without doubt the value of the glycemic index.

The glycemic index of foods is simply a ranking of foods based on their immediate effect on blood sugar levels. To make a fair comparison, all foods are compared with a reference food such as pure glucose and are tested in equivalent carbohydrate amounts.

Today we know the glycemic index of hundreds of different food items—both generic and name-brand—that have been tested following a standardized testing method. The table on pages 28 to 29 gives

the glycemic index of a range of common foods, including many tested at the University of Toronto and the University of Sydney. More
detailed tables are in Part III.

THE KEY IS THE RATE OF DIGESTION

Carbohydrate foods that break down quickly during digestion
have the highest glycemic index values. The blood glucose, or
sugar, response is fast and high. In other words the glucose in the
bloodstream increases rapidly. Conversely, carbohydrates which
break down slowly, releasing glucose gradually into the bloodstream, have low glycemic index values. An analogy might be the
popular fable of the tortoise and the hare. The hare, just like high
G.I. foods, speeds away full steam ahead but loses the race to the
tortoise with his slow and steady pace. Similarly, slow and steady
low G.I. foods produce a smooth blood sugar curve without wild
fluctuations.

For most people most of the time, the foods with a low glycemic
index have advantages over those with high G.I. values. But there are
some athletes who can benefit from the use of high G.I. foods during and after competition. This is covered in Chapter 6. The graph
on page 81 shows the effect of slow and fast carbohydrate on sugar
levels in the blood.

The substance which produces the greatest rise in blood sugar levels is pure glucose itself. All other foods have less effect when fed in
equal amounts of carbohydrate. The glycemic index of pure glucose
is set at 100, and every other food is ranked on a scale from 0 to 100
according to its actual effect on blood sugar levels.

The glycemic index of a food cannot be predicted from its composition or the glycemic index of related foods. To test the glycemic
index, you need real people and real foods. We describe how the
glycemic index of a food is measured on page 26. There is no easy,
inexpensive substitute test. Standardized methods are always followed so that results from one group of people can be directly compared with those of another group.

In total, eight to ten people need to be tested and the glycemic index of the food is the average value of the group. We know this average figure is reproducible and that a different group of volunteers will produce a similar result. Results obtained in a group of people with diabetes are comparable to those without diabetes.

The most important point to note is that all foods are tested in equivalent carbohydrate amounts. For example, 100 grams of bread (about 3½ slices of sandwich bread) is tested because this contains 50 grams of carbohydrate. Likewise, 60 grams of jelly beans (containing 50 grams of carbohydrate) is compared with the reference food. We know how much carbohydrate is in a food by consulting food composition tables, the manufacturer's data or measuring it ourselves in the laboratory.

THE GLYCEMIC INDEX IS A CLINICALLY

PROVEN TOOL IN ITS APPLICATIONS

TO DIABETES, APPETITE CONTROL, AND

REDUCING THE RISK OF HEART DISEASE.

HOW SCIENTISTS MEASURE THE GLYCEMIC INDEX

1. An amount of food containing 50 grams of carbohydrate is given to a volunteer to eat. For example, to test boiled spaghetti, the volunteer would be given 200 grams of spaghetti, which supplies 50 grams of carbohydrate (we work this out from food composition tables)—50 grams of carbohydrate is equivalent to 3 tablespoons of pure glucose powder.

2. Over the next two hours (or three hours if the volunteer has diabetes), we take a sample of their blood every 15 minutes during the first hour and thereafter every 30 minutes. The blood sugar level of these blood samples is measured in the laboratory and recorded.

3. The blood sugar level is plotted on a graph and the area under the curve is calculated using a computer program (Figure 1).

4. The volunteer's response to spaghetti (or whatever food is being tested) is compared with his or her blood sugar response to 50 grams of pure glucose (the reference food).

5. The reference food is tested on two or three separate occasions and an average value is calculated. This is done to reduce the effect of day-to-day variation in blood sugar responses.

6. The average G.I. found in 8 to 10 people is the G.I. of that food.

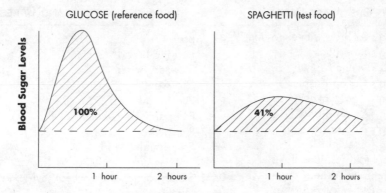

Figure 1. Measuring the glycemic index of a food. The effect of a food on blood sugar levels is calculated using the area under the curve (shaded area). The area under the curve after consumption of the test food is compared with the same area after the reference food (usually 50 grams of pure glucose or a 50 gram carbohydrate portion of white bread).

TODAY WE KNOW THE GLYCEMIC INDEX VALUES

OF HUNDREDS OF DIFFERENT FOOD ITEMS

THAT HAVE BEEN TESTED

FOLLOWING A STANDARDIZED METHOD.

THE GLYCEMIC INDEX OF SOME POPULAR FOODS

KEY

(Glucose = 100)
*Foods containing fat in excess of American Heart Associations guidelines
(av) Indicates that the G.I. is the average of several studies.

G.I. RANGES: The figures form a continuum, but in general:

LOW G.I. FOODS .... below 55
INTERMEDIATE G.I. FOODS .... between 55 and 70
HIGH G.I. FOODS .... more than 70

BREAKFAST CEREALS

Kellogg's All-Bran with extra fiber™	51
Kellogg's Bran Buds with Psyllium™	.45
Kellogg's Cocoa Krispies™	.77
Kellogg's Corn Flakes™	.84
Kellogg's Raisin Bran™*	.73
Kellogg's Rice Krispies™	.82
Kellogg's Special K™	.54
Oatmeal (old fashioned)	.49
Post Shredded Wheat™	.67
Quaker Puffed Wheat™	.67

GRAINS / PASTAS

Buckwheat groats	.54
Bulgur	.48
Rice	
Basmati	.58
brown	.55
long grain, white (av)	.56
short grain, white	.72
Uncle Ben's Converted™	.44
parboiled	.48
Noodles – instant	.46
Pasta	
egg fettuccine	.32
ravioli (meat)	.39
spaghetti (av)	.41
spirali	.43
Taco shells	.68

BREADS, MUFFINS, AND CAKES

Bagel	.72
Banana bread*	.47
Blueberry muffin*	.59
Croissant*	.67
Pita bread	.57
Pumpernickel (whole grain)	.51
Rye bread	.76
Sourdough bread	.52
Sponge cake	.46
Stoneground whole wheat (av)	.53
Waffles	.76
White bread (av)	.70
Whole wheat bread (av)	.69

CRACKERS / CRISPBREAD

Kavli™	.71
Crispbread	.81
Ryvita™	.69
Water cracker	.78

COOKIES

Arrowroot	.69
Graham crackers	.74
Oatmeal	.55
Shortbread*	.64
Social Tea™ biscuits	.55
Vanilla wafers	.77

VEGETABLES

Beets 64
Carrots 49
Parsnip 97
Peas (green) 48
Potato
   baked (av) 93
   new (av) 62
   red-skinned 88
   French fries 75
Pumpkin 75
Rutabaga 72
Sweet corn 55
Sweet potato 54
Yam 51

LEGUMES

Baked beans (av) 48
Broad beans (av) 79
Butter beans (av) 31
Chick peas (av) 33
Kidney beans (av) 27
Lentils (av) 30
Navy beans (av) 38
Soy beans (av) 18
Chana dal 8

FRUIT

Apple (av) 38
Apricot (dried) 31
Banana (av) 55
Cantaloupe 65
Cherries 22
Dates, dried 103
Grapefruit 25
Grapes 46
Kiwi 52
Mango 55
Orange (av) 44
Papaya 58
Peach – canned in juice 30
   fresh 42
Pear (av) 38
Pineapple 66
Plum 39

Raisins 64
Watermelon 72

DAIRY FOODS

Milk
   whole (av) 27
   skim 32
   chocolate flavored 34
Ice cream (av) 61
   low fat 50
Yogurt, flavored, low fat 33

BEVERAGES

Apple juice 40
Flavored syrup (diluted) 66
Fanta™ 68
Gatorade™ 78
Orange juice 46

SNACK FOODS

Corn chips* 72
Peanuts* 14
Popcorn 55
Potato chips* 54
Pretzels 83

SPORTS BARS

Power Bar™ Performance
   (chocolate) 58

CANDY

Chocolate* 49
Jelly beans 80
Life Savers™ 70
Mars Almond Bar* 68
Twix Cookie Bar™ 44
Snickers™ 41
Skittles Fruit Chews™ 70

SUGARS

Fructose 23
Glucose 100
Honey 58
Lactose 46
Maltose 105
Sucrose 65

GLUCOSE OR WHITE BREAD?

Some scientists have decided to use a 50 grams carbohydrate portion of white bread as the reference food because it is more physiological than glucose—typical of what we actually eat. On this scale, where the glycemic index of white bread is set as 100, some foods will have a G.I. value over 100 because their effect on blood sugar levels is higher than that of bread.

The use of two standards has caused confusion but it is possible to convert from one to the other using the factor 1.4 (100/70—white bread has a G.I. value of 70 when glucose is the reference food).

To avoid confusion throughout this book, we refer to all foods according to a standard where glucose equals 100.

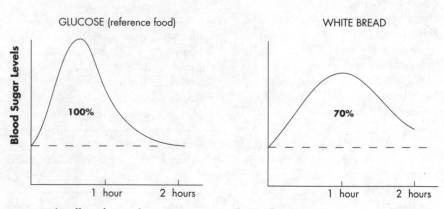

Figure 2. The effect of pure glucose (50 grams) and white bread (50 grams carbohydrate portion) on blood sugar levels.

The higher the glycemic index, the higher the blood sugar levels after consumption of the food. Foods with a high G.I. usually have a higher peak but a quicker fall and undershoot.

Rice Krispies (glycemic index equals 82) and baked potatoes (glycemic index equals 93) have very high glycemic index values, meaning their effect on blood sugar levels is almost as high as that of an equal amount of pure glucose (yes, you read it correctly). Figure 2 shows the blood sugar response to white bread compared with pure glucose. Foods with a low glycemic index (like lentils at

30) show a flatter blood sugar response when eaten, as shown in Figure 3. The peak blood sugar level is lower and the return to baseline levels is slower than with a high G.I. food.

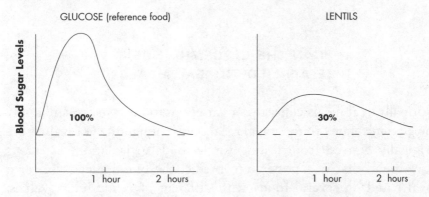

Figure 3. The effect of pure glucose (50 grams) and lentils (50 grams carbohydrate portion) on blood sugar levels.

WHY THE GLYCEMIC INDEX IS SO IMPORTANT

The slow digestion and gradual rise and fall in blood sugar responses after a low glycemic index food helps control blood sugar levels in people with diabetes. This effect may benefit healthy people as well because it reduces the secretion of the hormone insulin over the course of the day. Studies from Harvard University's School of Public Health show that diets with a low glycemic index are associated with a lower risk of developing type 2 diabetes and heart disease. Studies from the Children's Hospital in Boston show that overweight teenagers eat fewer calories on a low G.I. diet. (These issues are discussed in more detail in chapters 5, 7, and 9.) Slower digestion helps to delay hunger pangs and promote weight loss in overweight people. And recently, the United Nations WHO/FAO has recommended that all people base their diets on low glycemic index foods.

A food with a low glycemic index, eaten one to two hours before an event, gives the triathlete a winning edge by providing a slow-release source of fuel for the exercising muscles, thereby extending endurance. In contrast, a high glycemic index food given after the competition helps to restore muscle fuel stores faster, in good time for the next event.

These facts are not an exaggeration. They are not just preliminary findings. They are confirmed results of many studies published in prestigious scientific journals by scientists around the world.

CAN THE GLYCEMIC INDEX
BE APPLIED TO REAL MEALS?

Normally, real meals consist of a variety of foods. We can still apply the glycemic index to these real meals even though the G.I. values are originally derived from testing single foods in isolation. Scientists have found that it is possible to predict the blood sugar rise for a meal based on several foods with different glycemic index values. The total carbohydrate content of the meal and the contribution of each food to the total carbohydrate must be known. Data like this can be found in food composition tables.

For example, say you have a breakfast based on orange juice, cornflakes with milk and a slice of toast with a pat of butter. In the following table, you can see how the glycemic index of the total meal has been calculated. This may look complicated. In practice, people don't need to make these sorts of calculations at all. But dietitians and nutrition researchers sometimes have to. Many studies have shown a very close relationship between the predicted blood sugar response (as based on published glycemic index values of the relative effects of different foods and meals) and the actual observed blood sugar response.

■ ■ ■

HOW WE CALCULATE THE OVERALL GLYCEMIC INDEX OF A MEAL BASED ON SEVERAL FOODS WITH DIFFERENT G.I. VALUES

MIXED MEAL	CARBOHYDRATE (G)	% TOTAL CARBOHYDRATE	G.I.	CONTRIBUTION TO MEAL G.I.
Orange juice 4 ozs.	13	23	46	23% x 46 = 11
Kellogg's Corn Flakes™ 1 oz.	24	43	84	43% x 84 = 36
Milk 4 ozs.	6	11	27	11% x 27 = 3
1 slice of toast	13	23	70	23% x 70 = 16
Totals	**56**	**100**		**Meal G.I. = 66**

WHAT GIVES ONE FOOD A HIGH GLYCEMIC INDEX AND ANOTHER FOOD A LOW ONE?

Scientists have been studying what makes one food high and another low for more than fifteen years. There is a wealth of information that can easily confuse. We have summarized the results of their research in the following table which looks at the factors which influence the glycemic index of a food.

The key message is that the physical state of the starch in the food is by far the most important factor influencing the G.I. value. That's why the advances in food processing over the past two hundred years have had such a profound effect on the overall glycemic index of the food we eat.

■ ■ ■

FACTORS WHICH INFLUENCE THE GLYCEMIC INDEX OF A FOOD

FACTOR	MECHANISM	EXAMPLES OF FOOD WHERE EFFECT IS SEEN
Low degree of starch gelatinization	The less gelatinized (swollen) the starch, the slower the rate of digestion.	Spaghetti, oatmeal, cookies have less gelatinized starch
Physical form of food	The fibrous coat around beans and seeds and intact plant cell walls acts as a physical barrier, slowing down access of enzymes to the starch inside.	Pumpernickel and whole grain bread, legumes, barley, al dente pasta
High amylose to amylopectin ratio*	The more amylose a food contains, the lower its rate of starch digestion.	Basmati rice, legumes, cornstarch
Fiber	Viscous, soluble fibers increase the viscosity of the intestinal contents and this slows down the interaction between the starch and enzymes. Finely milled whole grain flours have fast rates of digestion and absorption because the fiber is not viscous.	Rolled oats, beans and lentils, apples
Sugar	The digestion of sugar produces only half as many glucose molecules as the same amount of starch (the other half is fructose). The presence of sugar also restricts gelatinization of the	Some cookies, some breakfast cereals

Factor	Mechanism	Examples of food where effect is seen
	starch by binding water during manufacture.	
Acidity	Acids in foods slow down gastric emptying, thereby slowing the rate of digestion.	Vinegar, lemon juice, salad dressings, acidic fruits, e.g. oranges, sourdough breads
Fat	Fat slows down the rate of stomach emptying thereby slowing the digestion of starch.	Potato chips have a lower glycemic index than baked potatoes

*Amylose and amylopectin are two different types of starch. Both are found in foods, but the ratio varies (see page 37).

The degree of starch gelatinization The starch in raw food is stored in hard compact granules that make it difficult to digest. This is why potatoes might give you a stomachache if you eat them raw. Most starchy foods need to be cooked for this reason. During cooking, water and heat expand the starch granules to different degrees, some granules actually bursting and freeing the individual starch molecules. This is what happens when you make a gravy by heating flour and water until the starch granules burst and the gravy thickens.

If most of the starch granules present have swollen and burst during cooking, the starch is said to be fully gelatinized. Figure 4 shows the difference between raw and cooked starch in potatoes.

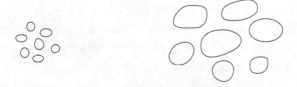

Figure 4. The difference between raw (compact granules) and cooked (swollen granules) starch in potatoes.

The swollen granules and free starch molecules are very easy to digest because the starch-digesting enzymes in the small intestine have a greater surface area to attack. The quick action of the enzymes results in a rapid and high blood sugar rise after consumption of the food (remember that starch is a string of glucose molecules). A food containing starch which is fully gelatinized will therefore have a very high glycemic index.

In foods such as cookies, the presence of sugar and fat and very little water, makes starch gelatinization more difficult, and only about half of the granules will be fully gelatinized. For this reason, cookies tend to have intermediate glycemic index values.

Particle size Another factor that influences starch gelatinization is the particle size of the food. Grinding or milling of cereals reduces the particle size and makes it easier for water to be absorbed and enzymes to attack. That is why cereal foods made from fine flours tend to have high glycemic index values. The larger the particle size, the lower the glycemic index as shown in Figure 5.

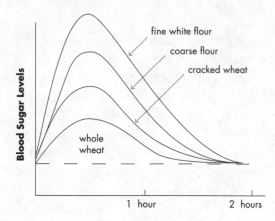

Figure 5. The larger the particle size, the lower the glycemic index.

One of the most significant alterations to our food supply came with the introduction of steel roller mills in the mid-nineteenth century. Not only did they make it easier to remove the fiber from cereal grains, the particle size of the starch was smaller than ever before. Prior to the nineteenth century, stone grinding produced quite coarse flours that resulted in slower rates of digestion and absorption.

When starch is consumed in its natural packaging—whole intact grains that have been softened by soaking and cooking—the food will have a low glycemic index. For example, cooked barley has a G.I. factor of only 25. Most cooked legumes have a glycemic index between 30 and 40. Cooked whole wheat has a glycemic index of 41.

The only whole (intact) grain food with a high glycemic index is rice, specifically low amylose rice. These varieties of rice have starch which is very easily gelatinized during cooking and therefore easily broken down by digestive enzymes. This may help explain why we sometimes feel hungry not long after rice-based meals. However, some varieties of rice have lower glycemic index values because they have a higher amylose content (see below) than normal rice. Their glycemic index values are in the range of 55 to 58.

Amylose and amylopectin There are two types of starch in food—amylose and amylopectin—and researchers have discovered that the ratio of one to the other has a powerful effect on the glycemic index of a food.

Amylose is a straight chain molecule, like a string of beads. These tend to line up in rows and form tight compact clumps that are harder to gelatinize and therefore digest (see Figure 6).

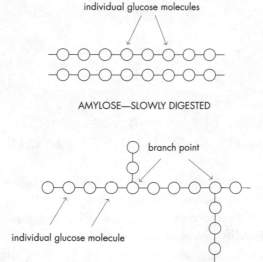

Figure 6. Amylose is a straight chain molecule which is harder to digest than amylopectin which has many branching points.

On the other hand, amylopectin is a string of glucose molecules with lots of branching points, such as you see in some types of seaweed. Amylopectin molecules are therefore larger and more open and the starch is easier to gelatinize and digest.

Thus foods that have little amylose and plenty of amylopectin in their starch have higher glycemic index values, e.g. wheat flour. Foods with a higher ratio of amylose to amylopectin have lower glycemic index values, including American long-grain rice, Basmati rice and all sorts of legumes.

WHY DOES PASTA HAVE A LOW GLYCEMIC INDEX?

The starting point for making pasta is semolina or cracked wheat, not wheat flour. Durum wheat makes the best pasta because the grain is extremely hard and the wheat breaks cleanly into distinct small pieces. The large particle size of semolina means that starch gelatinization is more difficult and thus enzyme attack is slowed down. The typical shape of pasta also appears to play a role in slowing down digestion. That's why pasta of any shape and size has a fairly low glycemic index (30 to 50). Cracked wheat and couscous used in Middle-Eastern cooking have intermediate glycemic index values.

HOW DOES THE GLYCEMIC INDEX
RELATE TO BLOOD INSULIN LEVELS?

Insulin is the hormone the pancreas produces to control blood sugar levels. (See "The Pancreas Produces Insulin" on page 4.) Insulin plays a vital role in maintaining good health. It is widely recognized that keeping insulin levels low in the blood is good for the body. High insulin levels are associated with weight gain, high blood fats, high blood pressure, and insulin resistance. Utilizing the glycemic index can help to regulate blood insulin levels because the insulin response to foods directly relates to the corresponding blood sugar response. The body converts the carbohydrate of low G.I. foods more slowly into glucose than it does high G.I. foods. Therefore, when you eat lower G.I. foods, less insulin is needed to bring the resulting small elevation in blood sugar under control. The higher the carbohydrate content of the diet, the more important it becomes to choose low G.I. foods.

THE EFFECT OF FAT AND PROTEIN
ON THE GLYCEMIC INDEX

High fat foods that have a low glycemic index may appear in a falsely favorable light because increases in fat and protein tend to slow the rate of stomach emptying and therefore the rate at which foods are digested in the small intestine. High fat foods will therefore tend to have lower glycemic index values than their low fat equivalents. For example, potato chips have a lower glycemic index (54) than potatoes baked without fat (85). Many sweet cookies have a lower glycemic index (55 to 65) than bread (70). But this is not a consistent finding. New boiled potatoes have a lower glycemic index (62) than French fries (75), despite the latter's fat content.

Remember, however, we need to eat a low fat diet, not a high fat one. So, high fat foods of any sort, whether low or high in their glycemic index, should only be eaten in limited amounts.

WHAT EFFECT DOES AN INCREASED CARBOHYDRATE
INTAKE HAVE ON BLOOD SUGAR LEVELS ?

While we know the G.I. of the foods is important, the total amount of carbohydrate in a meal must still be considered. As the amount of carbohydrate eaten in a meal increases (say from one to two to three slices of bread), the blood sugar response goes up as you might expect: Eating three slices of bread causes nearly three times the blood sugar response as one slice of bread. However, as more and more carbohydrate is eaten the blood sugar response does not increase indefinitely. In fact, eating six slices of bread causes only a slightly higher blood sugar response as eating three slices of bread.

However, blood insulin responses go up as carbohydrate intake increases. In fact, blood insulin responses go up and up and *up*, even though the blood sugar response does not. Thus, eating six slices of bread causes twice the insulin response as three slices, despite the fact that blood sugars vary minimally. Eating low G.I. foods *minimizes* the amount of insulin secreted when we eat a high carbohydrate diet.

A few scientists advise that high carbohydrate diets are not ideal because they make blood sugar and insulin levels go up. This is certainly true when high G.I. carbohydrates are chosen. However, large rises in blood sugar and insulin can be avoided by using lower G.I. foods. For example, if a dietitian advises that people with diabetes increase their carbohydrate intake from 60 g per meal to 80 g per meal, blood sugars would clearly be higher if they simply ate more of the same high G.I. foods. In theory the blood sugar response would go up by about 10 percent and the blood insulin by 20 percent. However, if lower G.I. foods were used instead, blood sugar and insulin might not go up at all. If low G.I. foods replaced all high G.I. foods in the diet, blood sugar and insulin would actually decline. That's the take-home message of this book.

THE EFFECT OF SUGAR ON THE GLYCEMIC INDEX

Table sugar or refined sugar (sucrose) has a glycemic index of only 60–65. This is because it is a disaccharide (double sugar) composed of one glucose molecule coupled to one fructose molecule. Fructose is absorbed and taken directly to the liver where much of it is slowly converted to glucose. So, the blood sugar response to pure fructose is very small (glycemic index of 23). Thus when we consume sucrose, in effect we have consumed only half as much glucose. This explains why the blood sugar response to 50 grams of sucrose is approximately half that of 50 grams of pure maltose (where the molecules are all glucose).

Many foods containing large amounts of refined sugar have glycemic index values close to 60. This is the average of glucose (G.I. = 100) and fructose (G.I. = 23). This is lower than that of ordinary soft bread with a glycemic index averaging around 70. Kellogg's

Cocoa Krispies which contain around 40 percent sugar have a glycemic index of 77, lower than that of Rice Krispies (82) which contain little sugar.

Another comparison of breakfast cereals is similarly instructive. Figure 7 shows the actual blood sugar responses after eating Golden Grahams compared to Team.

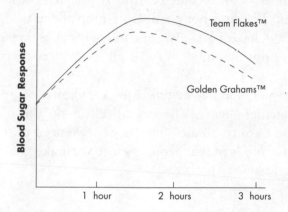

Figure 7. The blood sugar response of people with diabetes after eating General Mills Golden Grahams™ compared to Nabisco Team Flakes™.

Nearly half of the carbohydrate in Golden Grahams comes from sugar, whereas Team contains only a small amount of sugar. The reason for Team's higher blood sugar response is that it contains more refined starch, which has a higher G.I. factor than sugar. The lower blood sugar and lower blood insulin response of a cereal such as Golden Grahams applies even for people with diabetes. This does not mean that people should eat sugar indiscriminately. But it does mean there is no need to exclude all sugar from the diet.

So, contrary to popular opinion, most foods containing simple sugars do not raise blood sugar values any more than that of most complex starchy foods like bread. The same is true of honey (glycemic index of 58). Some types of honey have a much higher glycemic index (87) than refined sugar (65), possibly because they are a mixture of honey and glucose syrup.

Sugars that naturally occur in food include lactose, sucrose, glucose and fructose in variable proportions, depending on the food.

The overall blood sugar response to a food is very hard to predict on theoretical grounds because gastric emptying is slowed by increasing concentration of the sugars, whatever their structure.

Some fruits for example have a low glycemic index (grapefruit has a glycemic index of only 25) while others are relatively high (watermelon has a G.I. of 72). It seems the higher the acidity and osmotic strength (number of molecules per ml) of the fruit, the lower the glycemic index. Thus it is not possible to lump all fruits together and say that they will have a low glycemic index because they are high in fiber. They are not all equal. See the tables in Part III to compare fruits.

Many foods containing sugars are a mixture of refined and naturally occurring sugars. The overall effect on the blood sugar response is too hard to predict. This is why we need to test the G.I. value of sugary foods in real people before we make generalizations about their glycemic index.

THE EFFECT OF FIBER ON THE GLYCEMIC INDEX

The effect of fiber on the glycemic index of a food depends on the type of fiber. Finely ground cereal fiber, such as in whole wheat bread has no effect whatsoever on the rate of starch digestion and subsequent blood sugar response. Similarly, any cereal product made with whole wheat flour will have a glycemic index similar to that of its white counterpart. Breakfast cereals made with whole wheat flours will also tend to have high glycemic index values unless there are other influencing factors. Bran Flakes (74) and Weetabix (75), which are made from well cooked whole wheat grains, have high glycemic index values.

If the fiber is still intact it can act as a physical barrier to digestion and then the glycemic index will tend to be lower. This is one of the reasons why legumes have exceptionally low glycemic index values (30 to 40). It is also one of the reasons why whole (intact) grains usually have low glycemic index values.

Viscous fiber Viscous fiber thickens the viscosity or thickness of the mixture in the digestive tract. This slows the passage of food and restricts the movement of enzymes, thereby slowing digestion. The end result is a lower blood sugar response. Legumes contain high levels of viscous fiber, as do oats and psyllium (a seed which is a major ingredient in some breakfast cereals and laxatives). These foods all have low glycemic index values.

THE POWERFUL EFFECT OF ACID ON G.I. (VINEGAR, LEMON JUICE, SOURDOUGH BREADS)

Within the last few years, several reports in the scientific literature have indicated that a realistic amount of vinegar or lemon juice in the form of a salad dressing consumed with a mixed meal has significant blood sugar lowering effects.

As little as 4 teaspoons of vinegar in a vinaigrette dressing (4 teaspoons vinegar and 2 teaspoons oil) taken with an average meal lowered blood sugar by as much as 30 percent. These findings have important implications for people with diabetes or individuals at risk of diabetes, coronary heart disease or Syndrome X (impaired glucose tolerance, hypertension and high blood lipid levels).

The effect appears to be related to the acidity because other organic acids (such as lactic acid and propionic acid) also have a blood sugar lowering effect but the degree of reduction varies with the type of acid. Our findings show that among the various types of vinegar, red wine vinegar was the best. And lemon juice was just as powerful. It is well known that acidity in food puts the brake on stomach emptying slowing the delivery of food to the small intestine. Digestion of the carbohydrate in the food is therefore slowed and the final result is that blood sugar levels are significantly lower. Good news for people with diabetes! The take home message is that a side salad with your meal, especially a high G.I. meal, will help to keep blood sugar levels under control.

Sourdough breads, in which lactic acid and propionic acid are produced by the natural fermentation of starch and sugars by the yeast starter culture, also produce reduced levels of blood sugar and insulin compared with normal bread. The area under the plasma insulin curve was 22 percent lower with the sourdough product. In addition, there was higher satiety associated with breads having decreased rates of digestion and absorption. Thus there is significant potential to lower blood sugar and insulin and increase satiety with sourdough bread formulations.

CAN I MEASURE MY OWN
G.I. BLOOD SUGAR RESPONSE?

It is difficult for individuals to test the G.I. factor of a food themselves. People who normally monitor their blood sugar levels (for example, people with diabetes or hypoglycemia) may be tempted to compare their after-meal blood sugars with the published G.I. values and expect the two to match up perfectly.

While this may indeed be the case, it will not always be so. This is because the G.I. factor is based on the *overall* rise and fall in blood sugar. To compare two foods, you would need to measure blood sugar before you start to eat and several times over the course of the next three hours, particularly near the expected peak. The peak can occur at various times from 30 minutes to 3 hours (or 10 to 90 minutes in people without diabetes) after eating. You probably need to experiment to see when your blood sugar peaks—it will vary from food to food. Most people are not prepared to prick their fingers so frequently to draw blood for a glucometer!

And even then, you may not find a perfect match. This is because your blood sugar rise is not the same every day, even if you eat exactly the same thing. A blood sugar response after the same meal can vary by as much as 100 percent. Factors such as stress, time of day, recent exercise, health status (a headache, fever, or infection) and the length of time since the previous meal, can affect blood sugar responses. You can be reassured, however, that *on average* low G.I. foods will keep your blood sugar levels lower than high G.I. foods.

THERE IS NO NEED TO

EXCLUDE ALL SUGAR FROM THE DIET.

Chapter 4

THE GLYCEMIC INDEX AND YOU

YOUR QUESTIONS ANSWERED

*E*verybody can benefit from adopting the glycemic index approach to eating. It is the way nature intended us to eat. She packaged all the nutrients we needed in a slow-release form. Since the Industrial Revolution, however, we have taken nature's carbohydrates and manufactured them into fast-release or instant food as part of our quest for a more palatable, eye-catching and less perishable food supply. Unfortunately, the effect of all those instant foods is catching up on us in the form of diseases of affluence such as obesity and diabetes.

There is, however, no need to turn our backs on progress. We have sufficient knowledge of food and nutrition to let the pendulum swing back just enough to suit our needs. But we need the facts. We need answers. In this section we set out the facts about some of the most frequently asked questions about carbohydrates, diet and the glycemic index to dispel any lingering doubts.

Is it better to eat complex carbohydrate like starches instead of simple sugars?

There are really no big distinctions between sugars and starches in either nutritional terms or in the G.I. sense (see page 37). Some sugars such as fructose or fruit sugar have a low glycemic index. Others, such as glucose, have a high glycemic index. The most common sugar in our diet, ordinary table sugar (sucrose), has an intermediate glycemic index.

Starches can fall into both the high and low G.I. categories too, depending on the type of starch and what treatment it has received during cooking and processing. Most modern starchy foods, like bread, potatoes and breakfast cereals, contain high G.I. carbohydrate. What research has shown is that people with diabetes can eat the same amount of sugar as the average person, without compromising diabetes control. However, it is important to remember that sugar alone won't keep the engine running smoothly, so don't overdo it. Studies have shown that diets containing moderate amounts of refined sugars are perfectly healthy (10 to 12 percent of calorie intake) and the sugar helps to make many of the other nutritious foods in the diet more palatable.

THE SUGAR/FAT SEESAW

Did you know that fat and sugar tend to show a reciprocal or seesaw relationship in the diet? Studies over the past decade have found that diets high in sugar are lower in fat, especially saturated fat. Restricting sugar is frequently followed by higher fat consumption, and many fats are poor sources of nutrients. Thus a low sugar diet is not necessarily more nutritious. In some cases, high sugar diets have been found to have higher micronutrient contents, especially of calcium and riboflavin. This is because sugar is often used to sweeten some very nutritious foods, such as yogurts, breakfast cereals and milk. A low sugar (and high fat) diet has more proven disadvantages than a high sugar (and low fat) diet.

Are naturally occurring sugars in fruit better than refined sugar?

Naturally occurring sugars are those found in foods like fruit, vegetables and milk. Refined sugars are concentrated sources of sugar such as table sugar, honey or molasses. The rate of digestion and absorption of naturally occurring sugars is not different, on average, from that of refined sugars. There is wide variation within both food groups, depending on the food (see Figure 8). The glycemic index of fruits varies from 22 for cherries to 72 for watermelon. Similarly, among the foods containing refined sugars, some have a low glycemic index and some a high one. The glycemic index of sweetened yogurt is only 33, while a Mars Bar has a glycemic index of 65 (almost the same as bread).

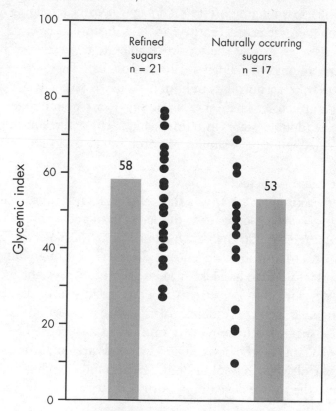

Figure 8. The figure shows the glycemic index values of foods containing either refined sugars or naturally occurring sugars (fruit, fruit juice etc.). The bars show the average value for each group. 'n' is the number of foods tested in each group.

Some nutritionists argue that naturally occurring sugars are better because they contain minerals and vitamins not found in refined sugar. However, new studies which have analyzed high sugar and low sugar diets have clearly shown that they contain similar amounts of micronutrients. People who eat lots of refined sugars tend to eat lots of food. Hence they eat more vitamins and minerals too.

Is honey better than sugar?

No, there is no benefit to substituting honey for sugar, unless you like the extra flavor that honey adds to a food. Both foods are concentrated sources of carbohydrate. Honey's glycemic index appears to be similar to that of refined sugar (about 60), unless the honey is glucose enriched (which increases its glycemic index). Honey was a major source of sweetness long before refined sugar became available at the beginning of the nineteenth century. In fact, historical research suggests that in some parts of the world people ate quantities of honey similar to the amount of refined sugar we now eat. There are negligible quantities of other nutrients in honey. Honey is basically a mixture of glucose and fructose. These two single sugars are bound together as a disaccharide (double sugar) in refined sugar. The end result of digestion in the small intestine is similar for both honey and sugar.

Does sugar cause diabetes?

No. There is absolute consensus that sugar does not cause diabetes. Type 1 diabetes (insulin-dependent diabetes) is an autoimmune health problem triggered by unknown environmental factors such as viruses. Type 2 diabetes (non-insulin dependent diabetes) is strongly inherited but lifestyle factors such as lack of exercise and overweight increase the risk of developing it. Because the dietary treatment of diabetes in the past involved strict avoidance of sugar, many people wrongly believed that sugar was in some way implicated as a cause of the disease. While sugar is off the hook, high G.I. foods are not. Studies from the Harvard University School of Public Health indicate that high G.I. diets increase the risk of developing both diabetes and heart disease.

Are rice and pasta equal as carbohydrates?

In the general sense that they are both high carbohydrate, low fat foods with valuable amounts of micronutrients, they are equal. Pasta has a higher protein content than rice but most people eat more than enough protein anyway. Pasta and rice are not equal in terms of the glycemic index values. The glycemic index of all types of pasta is low, usually between 40 and 50. Rice, however, can have a high G.I. (80 to 90) or a low G.I. (50 to 55) depending on the variety and, in particular, its amylose content (see page 32). In the U.S. many types of rice are available, and it is not always possible to identify the variety on the label. Waxy rice has a high glycemic index but Basmati, converted and parboiled rices appear to have low glycemic index values. The tables in Part III of this book (see pages 237 to 254) provide the glycemic index values of many types of rice.

What sort of variation do we see from day-to-day and between people?

Blood sugar responses show a certain degree of variability, both from day to day in the same person and between people. In non-diabetic subjects, the average day-to-day variation is 22 percent (i.e. the blood sugar response varies by an average of 22 percent). In people with type 2 diabetes, it is 16 percent, but in individuals with type 1 diabetes, it is as high as 30 percent. This means we should not expect to see precisely the same blood sugar levels after one particular food from one day to the next.

As is the case with any biological response there is quite wide variation between subjects—i.e., the blood sugar response in one person may be double that in another. However, it is clear that subjects tend to "track" well, giving high or low or intermediate responses on a consistent basis. In practice, therefore, foods will show the same ranking in terms of glycemic index in different subjects (see Figure 9).

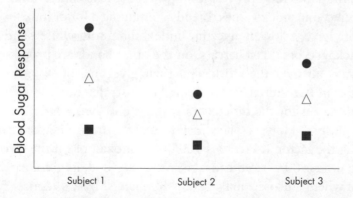

Figure 9. Three foods with high (●), intermediate (△) and low (■) glycemic index values will follow the same ranking in different individuals.

Why are there different G.I. values for the same food in different publications?

Different investigators testing the same food usually find close similarities in their G.I. values. For example, apples tested a glycemic index of 34 in one study and 40 in another. White bread tested 69 in one study, 71 in another. Don't be put off by such small differences. The glycemic index is an approximate result based on the average biological response of 10 or so people—and it's not as precise a measure as the carat weight of a diamond! In some instances (not too many, however), the differences in G.I. levels have been more marked; for instance, honey tested 58 in one study and 87 in another. While we can't be sure why this occurred, it is possible that the assumed carbohydrate content of the food was incorrect in one or other of the studies, leading to an under- or overestimation of the 50 gram carbohydrate portion used in glycemic index testing. Such a misestimation can markedly affect the final glycemic index result.

There may also be differences due to variations in the food itself. Rice is a good example of this. Genetically determined differences in the amylose content of rice means that different varieties of rice have very different glycemic index values. Basmati rice has a low glycemic index and waxy rice has a high glycemic index. In the early days of G.I. research, the variety of rice was not specified. Oats and oatmeal vary, too. To date we are not sure of the reasons for this. Potatoes vary with the variety and method of cooking. New or cocktail potatoes have lower G.I. values.

Again, the same food processed in different ways can produce very different glycemic index values. Breads containing a lot of intact whole grains will have a lower glycemic index than soft white sandwich bread. Packaged breakfast cereals, on the other hand, are processed in similar ways all over the world and their glycemic index values are very similar in the United States, Canada, Australia and elsewhere.

A third reason for the differences is the use of two reference foods, bread or glucose. However, it is easy to convert from one scale to the other using the factor 1.4 (equals 100/70). For example, if the glycemic index of a food is 80 when bread is the reference food, its glycemic index on a scale where glucose equals 100, is 80 divided by 1.4 (equals 57).

Is the glycemic index able to predict the effect of a mixed meal containing foods with very different glycemic index values?

Yes, the glycemic index can predict the relative effects of different mixed meals containing foods with very different glycemic index values. Over fifteen studies have looked at the glycemic index values of mixed meals. Twelve of these studies showed an excellent correlation between what was expected and what was actually found. You can predict the G.I. of a mixed meal by making a few simple calculations (see page 33).

The other three studies which did not show the expected correlation came from a particular group of researchers who were not using standardized methodology for working out the glycemic index from the area under the curve. In addition, their meals were high in fat instead of carbohydrate, and this tends to reduce the impact of any one carbohydrate food.

Won't the areas under the curve become equal (despite the different curves for a high and low G.I. food) if the testing is continued long enough?

Some people have assumed that the total area under the curve (for high and low G.I. food) will be the same if the blood sugar is simply measured for long enough. However, this is not the case because the body is able to restore normal blood sugar levels more quickly after a slowly digested food than a quickly digested one. An analogy is turning on a tap full force above a bucket with a small hole in the bottom of it. The bucket will fill up fast and empty slowly. In contrast, the same amount of water delivered as a slow trickle will empty with minimal accumulation (namely the area under the curve) in the bucket (see diagram on page 52).

Has the glycemic index been tested in long-term studies?

At least twelve studies to date have looked at the glycemic index in the diet in relation to long-term diabetes control. Some of these studies have been five weeks long, others, including ours, up to three months. All but one showed a clear benefit in improving blood sugar levels. People with high blood lipids (cholesterol, triglycerides) showed improvements in this area as well.

The insulin response is important and the glycemic index does not tell us anything about this. Is there a correlation?

In general, studies have found an excellent correlation between the

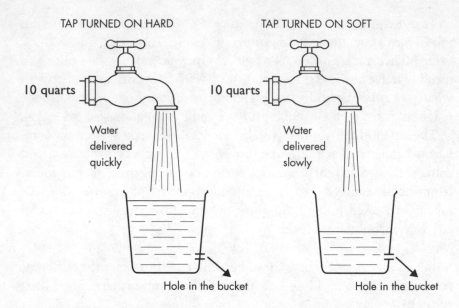

TAP TURNED ON HARD

TAP TURNED ON SOFT

10 quarts

10 quarts

Water delivered quickly

Water delivered slowly

Hole in the bucket

Hole in the bucket

Analogous to the high blood sugar
levels after a high G.I.food

Analogous to the low blood sugar
levels after a low G.I.food

glycemic index of a food and its insulin response. Sometimes the insulin response is higher or lower than expected. The presence of more protein will increase the insulin response proportionately. A large amount of fat may reduce the glycemic response but not the insulin response. But we should be avoiding large amounts of fat.

I'm confused about the G.I. of rice. Some people say it has a high glycemic index, others say it is low.

Rices in America usually have an intermediate or low glycemic index, probably because their amylose content is high. On page 32 we described how amylose is a form of starch which is more difficult to digest and results in lower glycemic index values. Long grain and converted rices sold in North America are high in amylose and have relatively low glycemic index values. You can guess at the glycemic index of rice by its appearance after cooking. If it is sticky and individual grains clump together, the rice is likely to have a high glycemic index. On the other hand, if the rice is dry and the grains separate, it is likely to have a relatively low glycemic index. There are many varieties of rice which show intermediate characteristics and therefore have intermediate G.I.s.

A high fat food may have a low glycemic index. Doesn't this give a falsely favorable impression of that food for people with diabetes?

Yes it does. The glycemic index of potato chips or French fries is lower than baked potatoes. The G.I. of corn chips is lower than sweet corn. It is important not to base your food choices on the glycemic index alone. It is essential to look at the fat content of foods as well. Low fat eating helps control weight, especially for people with diabetes.

What effect does fiber have on the G.I. value?

There is no simple answer to this question. Dietary fiber is not one chemical constituent like fat and protein. It is composed of many different sorts of molecules. Fiber can lower the glycemic index in some foods and not in others, depending on its physical form.

Soluble fiber tends to be viscous (thick and jelly-like) and can slow down digestion. Thus, the presence of soluble fiber in such foods as oats and legumes may contibute to their low glycemic index values. Purified psyllium added to foods slows down digestion because it is viscous.

Insoluble fiber in flours is finely ground and often doesn't slow digestion. Whole wheat bread and white bread have similar glycemic index values. Brown pasta and brown rice have similar values to their white counterparts. Sometimes insoluble fiber acts as a physical barrier which prevents the enzymes from attacking the starch. Whole (intact) grains of wheat, rye and barley have lower glycemic index values than cracked grains.

Are glycemic index values tested on healthy people valid for use in people with diabetes?

Yes, there are several studies which show a good correlation between values for the same foods obtained in healthy people and people with diabetes (type 1 and type 2). This is no surprise because the degree of glucose intolerance is allowed for in the calculation of the glycemic index.

Do low G.I. foods need to be eaten at every meal in order for people to see a benefit?

No, because the effect of a low G.I. food carries over to the next meal, reducing its glycemic impact. This applies even when the low G.I. meal is eaten for dinner. Its effect carries over to breakfast the following morning. But it is sensible to try to eat at least two low G.I. meals each day.

Bread has a G.I. of around 70 and lentils of around 30. Can I eat twice as much of the low G.I. food as the high G.I. food?

Yes, your blood sugar levels should be approximately the same after two servings of lentils or pasta compared with one serving of bread or potatoes. But you will have eaten twice as many calories. In practice, you will find that it is very difficult to eat a double portion of foods like lentils and pasta because they are very satiating and fill you up. If you can eat twice as much, it may be a good thing, because you are unlikely to have room for high-fat and less nutritious foods!

One study gave carrots a glycemic index of 95. Does this mean that a person with diabetes shouldn't eat carrots? What about other salad vegetables? And avocados?

The quantity of carrots that gives the 50 grams of carbohydrate portion (as used in standardized glycemic index testing) is enormous because they contain only about 7 percent carbohydrate. In fact, a 25 gram carbohydrate portion of carrots (about ¾ pound) were tested. This is much greater than the amount you would normally eat (about 3 ½ ounces).

Even with a glycemic index of 95, a normal serving of carrots would contribute only a small amount to the rise in blood sugar. Carrots and other foods like tomatoes, onions and salad vegetables that contain only a small amount of carbohydrate should be seen as "free" foods for people with diabetes.

Avocados are also insignificant sources of carbohydrate. Their glycemic index is effectively zero, and they therefore won't raise your blood sugar levels. They are rich in monounsaturated oils and many micronutrients, but unlike most other vegetables, they are also very high in fat and calories, so enjoy them in moderation.

If foods containing refined sugar have an intermediate glycemic index, does this mean that people with diabetes can eat as much sugar as they want?

Research has clearly shown that the glycemic index of refined sugar is the same in people who have diabetes and people who don't. Moderate consumption of sugar (which means 3–5 table-spoons of refined sugars a day) does not compromise blood sugar control. In fact, excluding sugar from the diet has important psychological consequences.

Sugar is not just empty calories, but a source of pleasure and reward and it helps to limit the intake of fatty foods and high G.I. carbohydrates.

Our advice is to spread your sugar budget over a variety of nutrient rich foods that become more palatable with the addition of sugar, e.g. yogurt, oatmeal and other breakfast cereals, jam on toast, milk drinks, and fruit desserts.

Bread and potatoes have high glycemic index values (70 to 80). Does this mean a person with diabetes should avoid bread and potatoes?

Potatoes and bread can play a major role in a high carbohydrate and low fat diet, even if a secondary goal is to reduce the overall G.I. factor. Only about half the carbohydrate has to be exchanged from high G.I. to low G.I. to achieve measurable improvements in diabetes control. So, there is still room for bread and potatoes. Of course, some types of bread and potatoes have a lower glycemic index than others and these should be preferred if the goal is to lower the G.I. as much as possible.

In the overall management of diabetes, the most important message is that the diet should be low in fat and high in carbohydrate. This will help people not only to lose weight, but to keep it off and improve their overall blood glucose and lipid control.

There are so few low G.I. foods that anyone wanting to follow a low G.I. diet would have to narrow the range of foods that he or she eats. Isn't this a bad thing?

It is a myth that you have to narrow the range of foods you eat on a low G.I. diet. In fact, some people have told us the opposite. They have found that the advent of the glycemic index has expanded the range of foods they can eat because foods containing sugar are not unduly restricted.

The rumor that all low G.I. foods are high in fiber and not very palatable also needs dispelling. It is true that legumes and All-Bran may not be everyone's favorite foods, but pasta, oats, fruit and many favorite Mediterranean recipes using cracked wheat and lentils etc. are low G.I. and delicious. To dispel such myths, we include many interesting, delicious recipes using legumes and lentils in Part II.

Does the area under the curve give a true picture of the blood sugar responses? Why not use just the peak value?

The area under the curve is thought to reflect the sum total of the glycemic response, not just the one time point given by the peak. Statisticians recommend use of the area under the curve. There is a very close relationship between the area under the curve and the peak response. That is, if one is high, the other is high and vice versa.

What about resistant starch? What effect does it have on the glycemic index of a food?

Resistant starch is the starch which completely resists digestion in the small intestine. It cannot contribute to the glycemic effect of the food because it is not absorbed. Resistant starch should not be included in the 50 gram carbohydrate helping which is the standard for G.I. testing because all of this 50 grams should be available carbohydrate, that is, available for absorption in the small intestine.

Resistant starch is not viscous like some forms of soluble fiber that delay absorption in the small intestine and flatten the blood glucose curve. Hence the mere presence of resistant starch in the food will not affect the glycemic index of a food. Bananas and potato salad both have relatively high amounts of resistant starch but the glycemic index values of these two foods are very different. Potatoes have a high glycemic index and bananas an intermediate one.

The difficulty that arises in testing is determining the true available carbohydrate content of food which is high in resistant starch. If some resistant starch is inadvertently counted as available carbohydrate in the 50 gram carbohydrate portion (e.g., 5 grams of the 50 grams), it will produce a falsely low glycemic index.

Does the glycemic index predict the glycemic effect of a normal serving of food?

Yes, studies have shown that even though the glycemic index has been determined on the basis of a 50 gram carbohydrate portion, it can be used to predict the effect of a normal serving size with a meal.

This is why the long-term studies of real people with diabetes eating real low G.I. meals have been successful.

Do people with diabetes need to reduce their insulin dose when they change to low G.I. foods?

It is possible that when people with well-controlled diabetes change their carbohydrate to low G.I. types that they could reduce their insulin dosage and maintain the same blood sugar levels. Doctors, dietitians, and nutritionists who have used the glycemic index in the management of diabetes report that some patients are eventually able to reduce their insulin dosages when a low G.I. diet is adopted. One study from Germany confirmed this in patients who used insulin pumps. Further scientific studies are needed to address the question in patients using ordinary injections of insulin.

Does the glycemic index of a food only apply to a certain quantity of the food?

No. The glycemic index of a food remains the same whether you eat 1 ounce of the food or 1 pound of the food. Because it is a ranking of one carbohydrate food to another according to glycemic impact, to make the comparison fair, the amount of each food being compared must be the same. This is why a 50 gram (usually) carbohydrate portion of a food is compared to 50 grams of glucose or a 50 gram carbohydrate portion of white bread, when the glycemic index is being measured. What does change with the quantity of food is the actual glycemic effect of that food in the body. We can eat less of a high G.I. food or more of a low G.I. food and end up with the same blood sugar responses.

Will the glycemic index be appearing on food labels?

In the United States, there are currently no plans to add information on the glycemic index to food labels. However, as the glycemic index becomes better known and understood, Americans will be increasingly interested in the G.I. levels of the foods they eat. At the same time, food manufacturers will respond to consumer demand by testing their foods and listing the glycemic index on food labels. In Europe, some breakfast cereal manufacturers already provide information on the back of cereal boxes about blood sugars, showing the differences between high G.I. and low G.I. foods. And in a first, in

early 1999 an Australian food company added information about
the glycemic index to the nutrition labels on their muffin product.

Can I still lose weight eating as much carbohydrate as I want?

Possibly not. We recommend a high carbohydrate intake and a
low fat intake. While carbohydrate is not usually stored as fat, if you
are eating more total energy than your body requires, then the carbohydrate will be used as a source of fuel in preference to fat. This
would have the effect of limiting the breakdown of body fat stores.
The idea is to eat enough energy in total to satisfy your appetite
(using low G.I. types helps) and nutritional requirements but not
more than you need. An increase in your activity level will help burn
up body fat as it is used as an additional fuel.

Why are there no glycemic index values for nuts and meats?

Nuts and meats contain little or no carbohydrate. Their glycemic
index is effectively zero, and when they are eaten by themselves, they
have negligible effects on blood sugar levels. Eaten with carbohydrates, nuts and meats help to slow down digestion and absorption
and reduce the glycemic index of a total meal. They are nutritious
foods that should be eaten in moderation, but nuts especially are
easy to overconsume, so watch how much you eat. Meat should
always be the leanest available and trimmed of excess fat.

Should I only eat foods with a low G.I.?

No, that is unnecessary. You can lower the G.I. of your diet effectively by substituting approximately half of your carbohydrate with
low G.I. types. When we eat a high G.I. food with a low G.I. food we
end up with a meal of intermediate G.I. so high G.I. foods needn't be
excluded. It is also generally healthier to eat as wide a variety of foods
as possible, so don't narrow your food choices unnecessarily.

EVERYBODY CAN BENEFIT FROM

ADOPTING THE GLYCEMIC INDEX APPROACH TO EATING.

IT IS THE WAY NATURE INTENDED US TO EAT.

Chapter 5

THE GLYCEMIC INDEX
AND WEIGHT LOSS

WHY IS BEING OVERWEIGHT A PROBLEM ANYWAY?

WHY DO PEOPLE BECOME OVERWEIGHT?

THE NEED FOR EXERCISE

WHAT FOODS CAUSE PEOPLE
TO BECOME OVERWEIGHT?

HOW CAN THE GLYCEMIC INDEX HELP?

YOU CAN CHECK YOUR DIET

KEEPING THE QUANTITY,
CUTTING BACK ON CALORIES

FOUR TIPS FOR PEOPLE TRYING TO LOSE WEIGHT

PLANNING LOW G.I. MEALS

*I*f you are overweight (or consider yourself overweight) chances are that you have looked at countless books, brochures and magazines offering a solution to losing weight. New diets or miracle weight loss solutions seem to appear all the time. They are clearly good for selling magazines, but for the majority of people who are overweight "diets" don't work (if they did, there wouldn't be so many!).

At best, (while you stick to it), a "diet" will reduce your caloric intake. At its worst, a "diet" will change your body composition. This is because many diets employ the technique of reducing your carbohydrate intake to bring about quick weight loss. The weight you lose, however, is mostly water (that was trapped or held with stored carbohydrate) and eventually muscle (as it is broken down to produce glucose). Once you return to your former way of eating, you regain a little bit more fat. With each desperate repetition of a diet you lose more muscle. Over years, the resultant change in body composition to less muscle and more fat makes it increasingly difficult to lose weight.

The real aim in losing weight is losing body fat. And perhaps it would be better described as "releasing" body fat. After all, to lose something suggests that we hope to find it again some day!

This chapter is not prescribing yet another "diet" for you to try. This chapter will give you some important facts about food and how your body uses it. Not all foods are equal. When it comes to what we eat and losing weight, it is not necessarily a matter of reducing how much you eat. Research in Australia and elsewhere has shown that **the type of food you give your body determines what it is going to burn and what it is going to store as body fat**. It has also revealed that certain foods are more satisfying to the appetite than others.

This is where the glycemic index plays a leading role. Low G.I. foods have two very special advantages for people who want to lose weight:

- they fill you up and keep you satisfied for longer,
- they help you burn more of your body fat and less of your body muscle.

Eating to lose weight with low G.I. foods is easier because you don't have to go hungry and what you end up with is true fat release.

WHY IS BEING OVERWEIGHT A PROBLEM ANYWAY?

If you are overweight you are at increased risk of a range of health problems. Among these are heart disease, diabetes, high blood pressure, gout, gallstones, sleep apnea (snoring) and arthritis. Along with this list of physical side effects of being overweight, there are an equal number of emotional and psychological problems.

Fifty-four percent of the adult American population is currently overweight, despite the expanding weight-loss industry and an ever increasing range of "diet," "lite," nonfat, and low fat foods. It is clear that the answer to preventing people from becoming overweight is not a simple one. Nor is losing weight easy to do. The glycemic index can make it easier, however. It tells you which foods satisfy hunger for longer and are the least likely to make you fat. When you use the glycemic index as the basis for your food choices:

- there is no need to overly restrict your food intake,
- there is no need to obsessively count calories,
- there is no need to starve yourself.

Learning which foods your body works best on is what using the glycemic index is all about.

It is worth taking control over aspects of your lifestyle that have an impact on your weight. You may not create a new body from your efforts, but you will feel better about the body you've got. Eating and exercising for your best performance is the aim of the game.

WHY DO PEOPLE BECOME OVERWEIGHT?

Is it genetic?
Is it hormonal?
Is it our environment?
Is it a psychological problem?
Or is it due to an abnormal metabolism?

Consider the energy balance paradox that exists in our bodies. For most of us, even without much conscious effort, our bodies maintain a constant weight. This is despite huge variations in how much we eat. For a proportion of people who are overweight this apparent balancing of energy intake and output seems lost or inoperative. So, despite every fad diet, every exercise program, even operations and medications, body weight can steadily increase over the years, regardless of all apparent efforts to control it.

It has always been said that our weight is a result of how much we take in and how much we burn up. So, if we take in too much (overeat) and don't burn up enough (don't exercise) we are likely to put on weight.

The question is: how much, of what, is too much?

The answer is not a simple one: not all foods that we eat are equal and no two bodies are the same.

People are overweight for many different reasons. Some people believe they only "have to look at food," others put on weight from "just walking past the bakery," others blame themselves because they eat too much. It is clear that a combination of social, genetic, dietary, metabolic, psychological (**and emotional**) factors combine to influence our weight.

"It must be in my genes." Before we talk more about food, let's look at the role genetics plays in weight control. There are many overweight people who tell us resignedly, that:

- "my mother's/father's the same,"
- "I've always been overweight,"
- "it must be in my genes."

Research shows us that this comment has much truth behind it. A child born to overweight parents is much more likely to be overweight than one whose parents were not overweight. It may sound like an excuse, but there is a lot of evidence to back the idea that our body weight and shape is at least partially determined by our genes.

Much of our knowledge in this area comes from studies in twins. Identical twins tend to be similar in body weight even if they are raised apart. Even twins adopted out as infants show the body-fat profile of their biological parents rather than that of their adoptive parents. These findings suggest that our genes are a stronger determinant of weight than our environment (which includes the food we eat).

It seems that information stored in our genes governs our tendency to store calories as either fat or as lean muscle tissue. Overfeeding a large group of identical twins confirmed that within each pair, weight gain was similar, however the amount of weight gained between sets of identical twins varied greatly. From this, researchers concluded that our genes control the way our bodies respond to overeating. Some sets of twins gained a lot of weight while others gained only a little, even though all were overconsuming an equivalent amount of calories.

MEASURING THE FUEL WE NEED

Calories are a measure of the fuel we need. Our bodies need a certain number of calories every day to work, just as a car needs so many gallons of gas to run for a day. Food and drink are our source of calories. If we eat and drink too much we may store the extra calories as body fat. If we consume fewer calories than we need, our bodies will break down its stores of fat to make up for the shortfall.

Metabolism   Our genetic make-up also underlies our **metabolism**, (basically how many calories we burn per minute). Bodies, like cars, differ in this regard. A V-8 consumes more fuel to run than a small 4-cylinder car. A bigger body, generally, requires more calories than a smaller one. Everybody has a **resting metabolic rate**. This is a measure of the amount of calories our bodies use when we are at rest. When a car is stationary, the engine idles—using just enough fuel to keep the motor running. When we are asleep, our engine keeps running (for example, our heart keeps beating) and we use a minimum number of calories. This is our resting metabolic rate. Our resting metabolic rate is the amount of calories we burn without any physical activity. When we start exercising, or even just moving around, the number of calories, or the amount of fuel we use, increases. However, the largest amount (around 70 percent) of the calories used in a 24-hour period are those used to maintain our basic body functioning.

Since our resting metabolic rate is how most of the calories we eat are used, it is a significant determinant of our body weight. The lower your resting energy expenditure the greater your risk of gaining weight and vice versa. We all know someone who appears to "eat like a horse" but is positively thin! Almost in awe we comment on their "fast metabolism," and we may not be far off the mark.

All this isn't to say that if your parents were overweight that you should resign yourself to being overweight. But it may help you understand why you have to watch your weight while other people seemingly don't have to watch theirs.

So, if you were born with a tendency to be overweight, why does it matter what you eat? The answer is that foods (or more correctly, nutrients) are not equal in their effect on body weight. In particular the way the body responds to dietary fat makes matters worse. **If you are overweight it is likely that the amount of fat you burn is small, relative to the amount of fat you store.** Consequently, the more fat you eat, the more fat you store. Although this may sound logical, the "eat-more, store-more" mechanism does not exist for all nutrients.

DID YOU KNOW?

The body loves to store fat. It is a way of protecting us in case of famine. In the midst of plenty we are building up our fat stores.

Among all four major sources of calories in food (protein, fat, carbohydrate and alcohol), fat is unique. When we increase our intake of protein, alcohol or carbohydrate the body's response is to **burn** more of that particular energy source. Sensibly, the body matches the supply of fuel with the type of fuel burned. One of the fundamental differences between fat and carbohydrate is that fat tends to be stored whereas carbohydrate has a tendency to be burned. It is worth noting at this point that if your carbohydrate intake is low, it may reduce the amount of calories you burn each day by 5 to 10 percent.

While you may not have been born owning the best set of genes, you can still influence your weight by the lifestyle choices you make. The message is simply this: if you believe that you are at risk of being overweight, you should think seriously about minimizing fat and eating more carbohydrate.

■ ■ ■

THE NEED FOR EXERCISE

A "fast metabolism" is not necessarily a matter of luck. Exercise, or any physical activity, speeds up our metabolic rate. By increasing our energy expenditure, exercise helps to balance our sometimes excessive caloric intake from food.

Exercise also makes our muscles better at using fat as a source of fuel. By improving the way insulin works, exercise increases the amount of fat we burn. A low G.I. diet has the same effect. Low G.I. foods reduce the amount of insulin we need which makes fat easier to burn and harder to store. Since body fat is what you want to get rid of when you lose weight, exercise in combination with a low G.I. diet makes a lot of sense!

WHY EXERCISE KEEPS YOU MOVING

The effect of exercise doesn't stop when you stop moving. People who exercise have higher metabolic rates and their bodies burn more calories per minute even when they are asleep!

WHAT FOODS CAUSE PEOPLE
TO BECOME OVERWEIGHT?

It was widely—and wrongly—believed for many years that sugar and starchy foods like potato, rice and pasta were the cause of obesity. Twenty years ago, every diet for weight loss advocated restriction of these carbohydrate-rich foods. One of the reasons for this carbohydrate restriction stemmed from the "instant results" of low carbohydrate diets. If your diet is very low in carbohydrate, you will lose weight. The problem is that what you primarily lose is fluid, and not fat. What's more, a low carbohydrate diet depletes the glycogen stores in the muscles, which makes exercise difficult and tiring.

Sugar has been blamed as a cause of people becoming overweight largely because it is often found in high fat foods, where it serves to make the fat more palatable and tempting. Cakes, cookies, chocolate and ice cream contain a mixture of sugar and fat. However, the primary sources of fat in our diet are **not** sweet. Fatty meat, cheese, French fries, potato chips, butter and margarine contain no sugar.

Current thinking is that there is little evidence to condemn sugar or starchy foods as the cause of people becoming overweight. Overweight people show a preference for fat-containing foods rather than a preference for foods high in sugar. In a survey performed at the University of Michigan where obese men and women listed their favorite foods, men listed mainly meats (protein-fat sources) and women listed mainly cakes, cookies, doughnuts (combinations of carbohydrate-fat sources). Other studies have found that obese people habitually consume a higher fat diet than people who have a healthy weight. So, it appears that a higher intake of fatty food is strongly related to the development of obesity—not carbohydrate-rich foods.

COUNTING THE CALORIES IN OUR NUTRIENTS

All foods contain calories. Often the calorie content of a food is considered a measure of how fattening it is. Of all the nutrients in food that we consume, carbohydrate—along with protein—yields the fewest calories per gram.

carbohydrate . . . . .4 calories per gram
protein. . . . . .4 calories per gram
alcohol . . . . .7 calories per gram
fat . . . . .9 calories per gram

Whether you are going to gain weight from eating a particular food really depends on how much that food adds to your total calorie intake in relation to how much you burn up. To lose weight you need to eat fewer calories and burn more calories. **If your total calorie balance does not change—there will be no change in your weight.** People who consume a high fat diet automatically eat a high calorie diet because there are more calories per gram in fatty foods. This is why eating low fat foods makes weight loss much easier.

HOW CAN THE GLYCEMIC INDEX HELP?

One of the hardest parts of trying to lose weight can be feeling hungry all the time, but this gnawing feeling is not necessary when you are losing weight. **Carbohydrates are natural appetite suppressants.** And of all carbohydrate foods, those with a low glycemic index are among the most filling and prevent hunger pangs for longer.

When we eat more carbohydrate, the body responds by increasing its production of glycogen. Glycogen is stored glucose, the critical fuel for our brain and muscles. The size of these stores is limited, and they must be continuously refilled by carbohydrate from the diet. Good glycogen stores ensure a well-fuelled body and make it easier to exercise.

In the past, it was believed that protein, fat and carbohydrate foods, taken in equal quantities, satisfy our appetite equally. We now know from recent research that the satiating (making us feel full) capacity of these three nutrients is not equal.

Fatty foods, in particular, have only a weak effect on satisfying appetite relative to the number of calories they provide. This has been demonstrated clearly in experimental situations where people are asked to eat until their appetite is satisfied. They over-consume calories if the foods they are offered are high in fat. When high carbohydrate and low fat foods are offered, they consume fewer calories, eating to appetite. So, carbohydrate foods are the best for satisfying our appetite without over satisfying our calorie requirement.

In studies conducted at the University of Sydney, people were given a range of individual foods that contained equal numbers of calories, then the satiety (that is, the feeling of fullness and satisfaction after eating) responses were compared. The researchers found that the most filling foods were foods high in carbohydrate that contained fewer calories per gram. This included potatoes, oatmeal, apples, oranges and pasta. **Eating more of these foods satisfies appetite without providing excess calories.** High fat foods that provide a lot of calories per gram, like croissants, chocolate and peanuts, were the least satisfying. These foods help us store more fat and are less filling to eat. Low G.I. foods are even more satiating than high G.I. foods. In fact, the lower the glycemic index, the more "replete" you'll feel.

Because fat is less satisfying to our appetite, it is easy to over-consume fatty calories. That is why reducing the dietary fat intake is a far more effective means of achieving weight control while satisfying the appetite than restricting carbohydrate intake. By eating a high carbohydrate diet it will be easier to lower your fat intake, and by choosing that carbohydrate from low G.I. foods, you make it even more satisfying.

What's more, even when the calorie intake is the same, people eating low G.I. foods may **lose more weight** than those eating high G.I. foods. In a study at Boston's Children's Hospital, the investigators divided overweight teenage boys into two groups: one group ate a low calorie, high G.I. diet and the other, a low calorie, low G.I. diet. The amount of calories, fat, protein, carbohydrate and fiber in the diet was the same for both groups. Only the glycemic index of the diets was different. The low G.I. group included foods like lentils, pasta, oatmeal and corn in their diet and excluded high G.I. foods like potato and white bread. After 12 weeks, the volunteers in the group eating low G.I. foods had lost, on average, 20 pounds—4 ½ pounds more than people in the group eating the diet of high G.I. foods.

How did the low G.I. diet work? The most significant finding was the different effects of the two diets on the level of insulin in the blood. Low G.I. foods resulted in lower levels of insulin circulating in the bloodstream. Insulin is a hormone that is not only involved in regulating blood sugar levels, it also plays a key part in when and how we store fat. High levels of insulin often exist in obese people, in those with high blood fat levels (either cholesterol or triglyceride) and those with heart disease. This study suggested that the low insulin responses associated with low G.I. foods helped the body to burn more fat.

WHICH FOODS ARE MOST FATTENING?

For the same amount of calories, you can eat far more carbohydrate food than fatty food. To prove the point, let's compare two everyday foods which are almost pure in the nutrition sense. Three teaspoons of sugar (almost pure carbohydrate) has the same number of calories as 1 teaspoon of oil (almost pure fat). This means that you can eat three times the volume of sugar as you could oil for the same calories!

Here are some examples of how you can eat more carbohydrate food than fatty food for about the same number of calories:

- A small grilled T-bone steak (about the size of a slice of bread) has the same calories as 3 medium potatoes.
- 3 slices of bread, thickly buttered, are equivalent to 6 slices of bread with no butter.
- 3 peanut butter cookies have more calories than a carton of low fat chocolate milk.
- Eating 1 piece of breaded, fried chicken at lunch substitutes for the calories of 6 slices of bread (without butter).
- For every 1 cup of fried rice you eat you could eat 2 cups of boiled rice.
- And if you're feeling extra hungry next time you stop for a coffee, consider that one slice of chocolate fudge cake has the calories of 4 slices of lightly buttered raisin toast!

In every case the highest fat foods have the highest calorie count. Because carbohydrate has about half the calories of fat, it is safer to eat more carbohydrate-rich food. What's more, the body will store fat and burn carbohydrate so the calories contribute more to your "spread" when they come from fat.

You can eat quantity—just consider the quality!

If you are still fearful of gaining weight from eating more pasta, bread and potatoes, consider this: the body actually has to use up calories to convert the carbohydrate we eat into body fat. The cost is 23 percent of the available calories—that is, nearly one-quarter of the calories of the carbohydrate are used up just storing it. Naturally, the body is not inclined to waste energy this way. In fact, the body converts carbohydrate to fat only under very unusual situations like forced overfeeding. The human body prefers the easy option. It is far more willing to add to our fat stores with the fat that we eat. Conversion of fat in food to body fat is an extremely efficient process and body fat stores are virtually limitless. No matter how excessive the amount of fat we eat, the body will always find space to store it.

No matter how excessive

the amount of fat we eat,

the body will always find

space to store it.

YOU CAN CHECK YOUR DIET

HOW MUCH CARBOHYDRATE DID YOU EAT YESTERDAY?

1. Recall the amounts of carbohydrate foods that you ate yesterday. Remember to include all those little snacks as well as the main meals!
2. Using the serving size guide below estimate the number of servings you had in the whole day. For example, if you had a banana, 2 slices of bread and a medium potato, this counts as 6 servings of carbohydrate.

Carbohydrate food	One serving is	How many did you eat?
Fruit	a handful or 1 medium piece	
Juice	about ¾ cup (6 ozs.)	
Dried fruit	¼ cup	
Bread	1 slice	
English muffin, bread roll, bagel	½ a roll, muffin or small bagel	
Crackers, crispbread	2 large pieces or	
	4–6 small crackers	
Rice cakes	2 rice cakes	
Muffin, cookies	½ a muffin or 2–3 cookies	
Sports bar/health bar	approximately ½ average bar	

Breakfast cereal	approximately 1 cup or 1 oz.
Oatmeal	about ¼ cup raw oats
Rice	½ cup of cooked rice
Pasta, noodles	½ cup of cooked noodles
Pancakes	about ½ a large pancake
Bulgur, couscous	about ½ cup, cooked
Potato, sweet potato	1 small potato, approximately 3 ozs.
Sweet corn	1 small cob or ½ cup kernels
Lentils	½ cup, cooked
Baked beans, other beans	about ½ cup, cooked
Total	

How did you rate?

Less than 4 servings a day	=	Poor.
Between 4 and 8 servings a day	=	Fair, but you need to eat a lot more.
Between 9 and 12 servings a day	=	Satisfactory, could do better.
Between 13 and 16 servings a day	=	Great.
Over 16 servings a day	=	You're a whiz!

IS YOUR DIET TOO HIGH IN FAT?

Use this fat counter to tally up how much fat your diet contains.

Circle all the foods that you could eat in a day, look at the serving size listed and multiply the grams of fat up or down to match your serving size. For example, with milk, if you estimate you might consume 2 cups of regular milk in a day, this supplies you with 16 grams of fat.

FOOD	FAT CONTENT (GRAMS)	HOW MUCH DID YOU EAT?
DAIRY FOODS		
Milk, (8 ozs.) 1 cup whole		

8

Food	Fat content (grams)	How much did you eat?
2 %	5	
skim	0	
Yogurt, 8 oz. container		
whole milk	7	
nonfat	0	
Ice cream, 2 scoops (1 cup)		
regular	15	
low fat	3	
fat free	0	
Cheese		
American, block cheese, 1 oz. slice	9	
reduced fat American cheese,		
1 oz. slice	7	
low fat slices (per slice)	3	
cottage, small curd, 2 tablespoons	3	
ricotta, whole milk, 2 tablespoons	2	
Cream, 1 tablespoon		
heavy	6	
light	5	
Sour cream, 1 tablespoon		
regular	3	
light	1	

FATS AND OILS

Butter, 1 teaspoon	4	
Oil, any type, 1 tablespoon (20 ml)	14	
Cooking spray, per spray	0	
Mayonnaise, 1 tablespoon	11	
Salad dressing, 1 tablespoon	6	

MEAT

Beef		
steak, flank, 3.5 ozs., lean only	10	
beef, ground, extra lean,1 cup		
(3.5 ozs.), cooked, drained	16	
sausage, frankfurter, grilled (2 ozs.)	16	

FOOD	FAT CONTENT (GRAMS)	HOW MUCH DID YOU EAT?
top sirloin, 3.5 ozs., lean only	8	
Lamb		
rib chop, grilled, lean only, 3.5 ozs.	10	
leg, roast meat, lean only, 3.5 ozs.	7	
loin chop, grilled, lean only, 3.5 ozs.	8	
Pork		
bacon, strips, panfried	9	
ham, 1 slice, leg, lean, 3.5 ozs.	5	
steak, lean only, 3.5 ozs.	4	
leg, roast meat, 3 slices, lean only, 3.5 ozs.	9	
loin chop, lean only, 3.5 ozs.	4	
Chicken		
breast, skinless, 3 ozs.	4	
drumstick, skinles, 2 ozs.	3	
thigh, skinless, 2 ozs.	6	
½ barbecue chicken (including skin)	30	
Fish		
grilled fish, 1 average fillet, 4 ozs.	1	
salmon, 3 ozs.	3	
fish sticks, frozen, 4 baked	14	
fish fillets, 2, batter-dipped, frozen, oven baked		
regular, 6 ozs.	26	
light	10	

SNACK FOODS

Chocolate bar, Hershey, 1.5 ozs.	13	
Potato chips, 1 oz.	10	
Corn chips, 1 oz. bag	10	
Peanuts, ½ cup (2.5 ozs.)	35	
French fries, 25 pieces	20	
Pizza, cheese, 2 slices, medium pizza	22	
Pie, apple, snack size	15	
Popcorn, fat and salt added, 3 cups	9	
Total		

How did you rate?

Less than 40 grams	=	Excellent.
		30 to 40 grams of fat per day is recommended for those trying to lose weight.
41 to 60 grams	=	Good.
		A fat intake in this range is recommended for most adult men and women.
61 to 80 grams	=	Acceptable.
		If you are very active, i.e. doing hard physical work or athletic training. It is too much if you are trying to lose weight.
More than 80 grams	=	You're possibly eating too much fat, unless of course you are Superman or Superwoman!

KEEPING THE QUANTITY, CUTTING BACK ON CALORIES

If you are trying to reduce your caloric intake there is still a **minimum** amount of certain foods that you should be eating each day. These are:

- **Breads/cereals/and grain foods—6 servings or more**
1 serving means   1 bowl breakfast cereal (1 oz.)
½ cup cooked pasta or rice
½ cup cooked grain such as barley or wheat
1 slice bread
½ small roll or muffin
- **Vegetables—3 servings**
1 serving means   1 small potato (about 3 ozs.)
Cooked vegetables such as broccoli or carrot—
½ cup
Raw leafy vegetables, such as lettuce—1 cup

- **Fruit—2-4 servings**
1 serving means: 1 medium orange (7 ozs.)
1 medium apple (5 ozs.)
½ cup strawberries

- Dairy foods—2 servings

1 serving means: 8 ozs. milk
                  1½ ozs. cheese
                  8 ozs. of low fat yogurt or other low fat dairy
                  foods

- Meat and alternatives—2 serving

1 serving means   2-3 ozs. cooked lean beef, veal, lamb or pork or
                  lean chicken (cooked weight,
                      excluding bone), skin removed
                  2-3 ozs. fish (cooked weight, excluding bone)
                  1 egg
                  ½ cup cooked lentils or dried peas or beans

In our experience, looking at the diets of hundreds of people who want to lose weight, the change required is often to **eat more!**

FOUR TIPS FOR PEOPLE TRYING TO LOSE WEIGHT

1. Eat regular meals—include snacks in between if you are hungry.

2. Try to include a low G.I. food at every meal.

3. Ensure that your meals contain mainly carbohydrate and only a little fat.

4. Eat low carbohydrate foods such as carrots, broccoli and salads freely, but don't eat them instead of the high carbohydrate foods.

PLANNING LOW G.I. MEALS

Breakfast
- Start with a bowl of low G.I. cereal served with skim or 1% milk or yogurt.
- Try something like All-Bran, or rolled oats (raw or cooked).
- If you prefer muesli or granola, keep to a small bowl of a low fat version—check that it doesn't contain added fats.

- Add a slice of toast made from 100% stoneground whole wheat bread or whole grain pumpernickel (or 2 slices for a bigger person) with a tablespoon of jam, sliced banana, honey, marmalade, or light cream cheese with sliced apple. Keep butter to a minimum, or use none at all.
- If you like a hot breakfast, try a boiled or poached egg with your toast.

Lunch

- Try a sandwich or roll, with only a dab of butter. Choose 100% stoneground whole wheat or whole grain pumpernickel, or any other bread made with lots of whole grains. Add plenty of sliced vegetables.
- For the filling choose from a thin slice of ham, pastrami, lean roast beef or chicken or turkey breast, or a slice of low fat cheese, salmon or tuna (in water), or an egg. An extra container of salad or vegetable soup will help to fill you up.
- Finish your lunch with a piece of fruit, or fruit salad with a low fat yogurt, or a low fat flavored or plain milk.

Dinner

- The basis of dinner should be high carbohydrate grains and root vegetables.
- Eat as many vegetables as you can, using a small amount of meat, chicken or fish.
- Use lean meat like top round beef, veal, pork, trimmed lamb, chicken breast, fish fillets, turkey. Red meat is a valuable source of iron—just choose lean types. A piece of meat, chicken or fish that fits in the palm of your hand (no fingers) fulfills the daily protein requirements of an adult.
- If you prefer not to eat meat, a cup of cooked dried peas, beans, lentils or chick peas can provide protein and iron without any fat. At the same time they supply low G.I. carbohydrate and fiber.
- Tofu and peanuts are good meat alternatives.
- Boost your fruit intake and get into the habit of finishing your meal with fruit—fresh, stewed or baked—or try a fruit sorbet.

Snacks

- It is important to include a couple of dairy food servings each day for your calcium needs. If you haven't used yogurt or cheese in any meals, you may choose to make a low fat milkshake. One or two scoops of low fat ice cream or pudding can also contribute to daily calcium intake.

- If you like whole grain breads, an extra slice makes a very good choice for a snack. Other snacks can include toasted sourdough English muffin halves, or half a bagel.

- Fruit is always a low calorie option for snacks. You should aim to consume at least 3 servings a day. It may be helpful to prepare fruit in advance to make it accessible and easy to eat.

- Low fat crackers (like water crackers) are a low calorie snack if you want something dry and crunchy, although they may not be as sustaining as a grainy bread. Popcorn (home prepared with a minimum of fat) is another good alternative.

- Keep vegetables (like celery and carrot sticks, radishes, jicama, baby tomatoes, florets of blanched cauliflower or broccoli) readily prepared to snack on, too.

IN OUR EXPERIENCE OF

LOOKING AT THE DIETS OF PEOPLE

WHO WANT TO LOSE WEIGHT,

THE CHANGE REQUIRED IS OFTEN TO EAT MORE.

Chapter 6

THE GLYCEMIC INDEX AND PEAK ATHLETIC PERFORMANCE

WHY IS THE GLYCEMIC INDEX RELEVANT
TO ATHLETIC PERFORMANCE?

A HIGH CARBOHYDRATE DIET IS ESSENTIAL
FOR PEAK ATHLETIC PERFORMANCE

MISCONCEPTIONS ABOUT CARBOHYDRATES

THE CASE FOR LOW G.I. FOODS

THE PRE-EVENT MEAL

THE CASE FOR HIGH G.I. FOODS

DURING AN EVENT

RECOVERY (AFTER THE EVENT)

HOW MUCH FOOD DO YOU NEED TO EAT
TO GET THIS MUCH CARBOHYDRATE?

THE TRAINING DIET AND
CARBOHYDRATE LOADING

HOW DO YOU CHOOSE A HIGH
CARBOHYDRATE DIET?

IS YOUR DIET FIT FOR PEAK PERFORMANCE?

*A*ustralian scientists were the first in the world to apply the concept of the glycemic index to athletics and exercise. Canadian scientists "invented" the G.I. approach to help classify carbohydrates but Australian researchers could see that what they were doing had important implications for athletic performance. Recent research in the United States has confirmed the Australian findings. Manipulating the G.I. of the diet can give you the winning edge—whether you are one of the elite or a weekend warrior.

WHY IS THE GLYCEMIC INDEX RELEVANT TO ATHLETIC PERFORMANCE?

The glycemic index ranks foods on the basis of their measured blood sugar response. The rate at which glucose enters the bloodstream affects the insulin response to that food and ultimately affects the fuels available to the exercising muscles. There are times when low G.I. foods provide an advantage and times when high G.I. foods are better. For best performance, a serious athlete needs to learn about which foods have high and low glycemic index values and when to eat them.

High glycemic index foods like potatoes will produce a rapid increase in glucose and insulin levels, something which is not desirable just before a race when glycogen stores should already be fully charged. Low G.I. foods, such as pasta, which are digested and absorbed much more slowly, are able to provide glucose to the working muscle towards the end of exercise when glycogen stores are running low. They can be likened to a continuous injection of glucose during the event. This can boost energy when fatigue begins to set in. After the event, high G.I. foods are best because they stimulate more insulin, the hormone responsible for putting glycogen back into the muscles.

MANIPULATING THE G.I.

OF YOUR DIET CAN GIVE YOU

THE WINNING EDGE!

A HIGH CARBOHYDRATE DIET IS ESSENTIAL FOR PEAK ATHLETIC PERFORMANCE

A high carbohydrate diet is a must for optimum athletic performance because it produces the biggest stores of muscle glycogen. As we have previously described, the carbohydrate we eat is stored in the body in the form of glycogen in the muscles and liver. A small amount of carbohydrate (about 1 teaspoon) circulates as glucose in the blood. When you are exercising at a high intensity, your muscles rely on glycogen and glucose for fuel. Although the body can use fat when exercising at lower intensities, fat cannot provide the fuel fast enough when you are working very hard. The bigger your stores of glycogen and glucose, the longer you can go before fatigue sets in.

Unlike the fat stores in the body which can release almost unlimited amounts of fatty acids, the carbohydrate stores are small. They are fully depleted after two or three hours of strenuous exercise. This drying up of carbohydrate stores is often called **"hitting the wall."** The blood glucose concentration begins to decline at this point. If exercise continues at the same rate, blood glucose may drop to levels which interfere with brain function and cause disorientation and unconsciousness. Some athletes refer to this as a "hypo" and in cycling it is known as "bonking."

All else being equal, the eventual winner is the person with the largest stores of muscle glycogen. Any good book on nutrition for athletes will tell you how to maximize your muscle glycogen stores by ingesting a high carbohydrate training diet and by "carbohydrate loading" in the days prior to the competition. In this chapter we provide instructions for increasing muscle glycogen as well as using the glycemic index to your advantage in sport.

MISCONCEPTIONS ABOUT CARBOHYDRATES

Many athletes and coaches have misconceptions about carbohydrates that can affect athletic performance. In the past we were taught that simple carbohydrates (sugars) were digested and absorbed rapidly while complex carbohydrates (starches) were digested slowly. We assumed (completely incorrectly) that simple carbohydrates gave the most rapid rises in blood sugar while complex carbohydrates produced gradual rises. Unfortunately, these assumptions had no factual or scientific basis. They were based on structural considerations, smaller molecules, like sugars, being thought to be easier to digest than larger ones, like starches. Even though incorrect, the logical nature of these assumptions meant that they were rarely ever questioned. Unfortunately, many people still think sugars are the best source of quick energy and that starches are our best source of sustained energy.

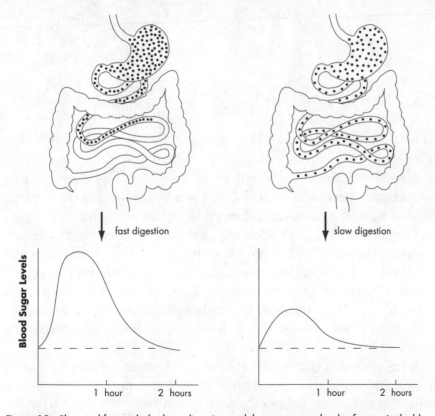

Figure 10. Slow and fast carbohydrate digestion and the consequent levels of sugar in the blood

THE CASE FOR LOW G.I. FOODS

Imagine that it is possible to carry a hidden reservoir or an extra store of carbohydrate to use when needed. It must be in the small intestine, not the stomach where it may cause nausea during the event.

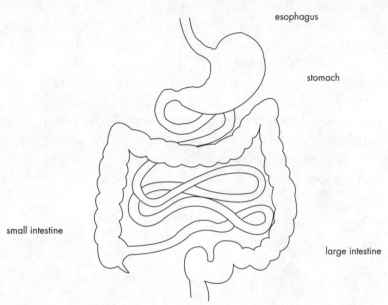

esophagus

stomach

small intestine

large intestine

Figure 11. The gastrointestinal tract of the human body.

A meal containing carbohydrate is best eaten about one to two hours before strenuous exercise, such as a race, allowing time for the food to leave the stomach and reach the small intestine.

The problem is that by allowing a gap of about two hours, the carbohydrate in most foods would have been burned up well before the race begins. The small intestine would be empty and no longer acting as a reservoir of carbohydrate. There is one other possibility. What if you could package the carbohydrate in such a way as to make it be released more slowly from the small intestine during the event?

What is needed is a food that is so slowly digested that it remains in the small intestine for hours after consumption. Only some foods have their carbohydrate packaged in such a way as to make it slowly digested and absorbed and gradually released from the small intestine. In the same way that certain drugs have been formulated as **lente** (the Italian word for **slowly**) or "slow-release" compounds so that the drug's action is evenly maintained throughout the day, it is possible to do this with the carbohydrate in food, too.

It shouldn't come as a surprise to learn that nature originally provided carbohydrate in a slow-release form or as lente carbohydrate. Starch and sugars in raw, unprocessed foods are packaged in a cell matrix surrounded by fiber and only gradually broken down by the enzymes of the gastrointestinal tract. In the days of hunter-gatherers, when early humans literally ran for their lives from predatory animals, slow-release carbohydrate gave them the ultimate survival advantage. Before the introduction of horses, American Indians ran for miles rounding up bison and herding them over the cliffs to their death. The traditional foods of these people provided a slow-release source of glucose for the exercising muscle.

Fortunately, there are still some foods in our modern diet that remain slowly digested and absorbed. These foods have a glycemic index less than 55. They include all kinds of pasta, barley, whole grains, oatmeal, All-Bran and some varieties of rice, and bread made with softened whole grains. They also include many foods made with lentils, chick peas, couscous and barley. The traditional Mediterranean diet is high in legumes, which have exceptionally low glycemic index values.

Low G.I. foods have been proven by both American and Australian researchers to extend endurance when eaten alone one to two hours before prolonged strenuous exercise. When a pre-event meal of lentils (low glycemic index) was compared with one of potatoes (high glycemic index), cyclists were able to continue cycling at high intensity (65 percent of their maximum) for 20 minutes longer when the meal was lentils. Their blood sugar and insulin levels were significantly higher at the end of exercise, indicating that carbohydrate was still being absorbed from the small intestine even after 90 minutes of strenuous exercise. Figure 12 shows the blood sugar levels during exercise after consumption of low and high G.I. foods.

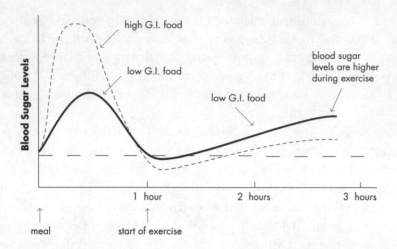

Figure 12. Comparison of the effect of low and high G.I. foods on blood sugar levels during prolonged strenuous exercise.

THE PRE-EVENT MEAL

Before you read any further, it's important to appreciate the type of event where the glycemic index will help. It is one in which the athlete is undertaking a very strenuous form of exercise for longer than 90 minutes. Exercise physiologists define this by saying that the athlete is exercising at more than 65 percent of their maximum capacity for a prolonged period. Examples of such events include a running or swimming marathon, a triathlon, non-stop tennis competition or soccer game (depending on the player's position). Some forms of recreation such as cross-country skiing and mountain climbing may also benefit from the G.I. approach. In some occupations that require prolonged strenuous activity for hours and hours (such as forest fire-fighting), low G.I. foods may be beneficial.

Low G.I. foods are best before an event—approximately two hours before the big race. The meal will have left the stomach by then but continues to be digested in the small intestine for hours afterwards. The slow rate of carbohydrate digestion in low G.I. foods helps ensure that a steady stream of glucose is released into the bloodstream during the event. The extra glucose is available when needed towards the end of the exercise when muscle carbohydrate stores are running low. In this way, low G.I. foods increase endurance and prolong the time before exhaustion hits.

It's also important to select low G.I. foods that do not cause gastrointestinal discomfort such as stomach cramps and flatulence. Some low G.I. foods such as legumes are high in fiber or indigestible sugars. However, not all low G.I. foods are fibrous and high residue. The high amylose rices (e.g. Basmati) and any form of white pasta are good examples of low G.I. foods that don't contain much fiber. Instant noodles have a low G.I., too. Athletes who are too nervous to eat a solid meal may prefer a milk-based supplement such as Exceed.

EVENTS WHERE THE GLYCEMIC INDEX CAN GIVE YOU THE EDGE

running marathon

swimming marathon

triathlon

non-stop tennis competition

soccer game (depending on the player's position)

cross-country skiing

mountain climbing

prolonged strenuous aerobics and gym work-outs (longer than 90 minutes)

The food industry is increasingly interested in the glycemic index, too, and it won't be long before there are specially formulated low G.I. foods on the supermarket shelves specifically aimed at the serious athlete. The sports drinks that have become popular have a high glycemic index, between 70 and 80. So they may not be an advantage before the event, but they are an invaluable aid during the event when blood sugar needs to be topped up, as well as after the event when glycogen stores need to be replenished.

■ ■ ■

THE PRE-EVENT MEAL

How much should I eat before the event?

About 1 gram of carbohydrate for each 2.2 lbs. of body weight (i.e. 50 grams of carbohydrate if you weigh 110 lbs., or 75 grams of carbohydrate if you weigh 165 lbs.)

How soon before?

1 to 2 hours before the event is a good starting point.
You should experiment to determine the timing that works best for you.

The following table shows the serving sizes of low G.I. foods containing 50 grams or 75 grams of carbohydrate.

You will not win if your pre-event meal is jiggling around in your stomach (this will affect the jogger more than the cyclist). So test the timing and amount of low G.I. food during your training sessions. Then you'll be ready for the big day. Don't try it out for the first time on the day of the competition!

■ ■ ■

SERVING SIZES OF LOW G.I. FOODS TO EAT
1 TO 2 HOURS BEFORE THE EVENT

FOOD	GLYCEMIC INDEX	SERVING SIZE = 50 G CARBOHYDRATE	SERVING SIZE = 75 G CARBOHYDRATE
Heavy grain breads Pumpernickel bread,	41	3 slices (approx 3 ozs.)	4 to 5 slices (approx 5 ozs.)
Spaghetti, cooked	37	1½ cups (6 ozs.)	2¼ cups (10 ozs.)
Oatmeal, cooked	49	2½ cups (20 ozs.)	3½ cups (32 ozs.)
Baked beans	48	medium can (16 ozs.)	1½ medium cans (24 ozs.)
Fruit salad	approx 50	2½ cups (approx 16 ozs.)	4 cups (28 ozs.)
Yogurt (low fat)	33	2 containers (16 ozs.)	3 containers (24 ozs.)
Apples	38	3 small medium (16 ozs.)	4 small (20 ozs.)
Oranges	44	5 small (20 ozs.)	7 small (32 ozs.)
Dried apricots	31	¾ cup (4 ozs.)	1⅓ cups (4 ozs.)

Females weighing about 110 lbs. should aim to eat 50 grams of carbohydrate.
Males weighing about 165 lbs. should aim to eat 75 grams of carbohydrate.

THE CASE FOR HIGH G.I. FOODS

The pre-event meal should be low G.I., but at other times, high G.I. foods are preferable. This includes during the event, after the event and after normal training sessions. This is because high G.I. foods are digested and absorbed faster and stimulate more insulin, the hormone responsible for getting glucose into the muscles for either immediate or future use.

■ ■ ■

DURING AN EVENT

High G.I. foods should be used during events lasting longer than 90 minutes. This form of carbohydrate is rapidly released into the bloodstream and ensures that glucose is available for oxidation in the muscle cells. Liquid foods are usually tolerated better than solid foods while racing because they are emptied more quickly from the stomach. Sports drinks are ideal during the race because they replace water and electrolytes as well. The old standby of bananas strapped to the bike doesn't have much scientific basis unless they are very ripe. The G.I. of bananas is only 55 and some of their carbohydrate is completely resistant to digestion (which could give you gas and a stomachache). If you feel hungry for something solid during a cycling race, try jelly beans (G.I. of 80), dried dates or sports bars containing high amounts of glucose and maltodextrins.

USING THE G.I. FACTOR ON THE DAY OF THE EVENT

LOW G.I. • BREAKFAST
Large bowl of oatmeal with low fat milk
Pasta with tomato-based sauce
Juice
Fruit (apple, orange juice, kiwi, canned
    peaches or pears)
Cereal (All-Bran™, oats)
Whole grain bread, toasted with jam
    or honey

HIGH G.I. SNACK • DURING THE EVENT
(aim for 30 g carbohydrate and 16
    ozs. water per hour) e.g. at least
    16 ozs. sports drink
or 12 jelly beans + at least 16 ozs.
    water
or honey sandwich + at least 16 ozs.
    water

LOW G.I. SNACK • 1–2 HOURS PRE-EVENT
Dried apricots
Sports bars
Fruit smoothie made with any low G.I.
    fruit and low fat milk
Whole grain bread, toasted or
    sandwiches
Fruit salad and yogurt
Pasta with low fat sauce

HIGH G.I. SNACK • AFTER THE EVENT (WITHIN 30–60 MINUTES)
32 ozs. of sports drink or Gatorade™
or ½ cup creamed rice
or 6–8 dried dates
or bowl of Rice Krispies™ or corn
    flakes

INTERMEDIATE G.I. • DINNER
2 cups of rice with meat or tuna
Vegetables—carrots, broccoli etc.
2 slices bread

2 cups of fruit salad and 8 oz.
container of yogurt

CONSUME **30** TO **60** GRAMS OF CARBOHYDRATE

PER HOUR DURING THE EVENT.

RECOVERY (AFTER THE EVENT)

In some competitive sports, athletes compete on consecutive days and glycogen stores need to be at their maximum each time. Here it is important to restock the glycogen store in the muscles as fast as possible after the event. High G.I. foods are best in this situation. Sports scientists at the Australian Institute of Sport in Canberra have shown that high G.I. foods resulted in faster replenishment of glycogen into the fatigued muscles (see Figure 13). Muscles are more sensitive to glucose in the bloodstream in the first hour after exercise, so a concerted effort should be made to get as many high G.I. foods in as soon as possible.

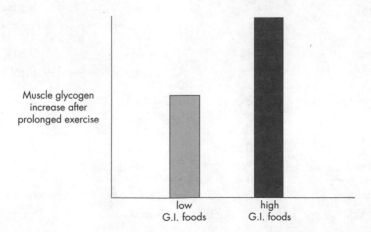

Figure 13. Comparison of the effect of low and high G.I. foods on replenishment of muscle glycogen levels after exercise.

Suggested foods include most of the sports drinks on the market (which replace water and electrolyte losses too), or instant potatoes, breads and breakfast cereals with a high G.I. such as cornflakes and Rice Krispies. Soft drinks have an intermediate G.I., so they won't be ideal but they won't do any harm either. The table below shows the high G.I. foods that are best after and between exercise workouts.

SERVING SIZES OF HIGH G.I. FOODS TO EAT DURING AND AFTER EVENTS

FOOD	G.I.	SERVING SIZE = 50 GRAMS CARBOHYDRATE	SERVING SIZE = 75 GRAMS CARBOHYDRATE
White or brown bread	70	approx 3 ozs. (3 slices)	approx 5 ozs. (4–5 slices)
Rice Krispies™	82	1 ½ ozs. (1½ cups) + 6 ozs. low fat milk	2 ⅓ ozs. (2 cups) + 10½ ozs. milk
Kellogg's Corn Flakes™	84	1 ½ ozs. (1½ cups) + 6 ozs. low fat milk	2 ⅓ ozs. (2 cups) + 10 ½ ozs. milk
Rice cakes	82	2 ozs. (5 rice cakes)	3 ozs. (8 rice cakes)
Crispbread	81	2 ⅓ ozs. (13 crispbread)	3 ozs. (19 crispbread)
Water crackers	78	2 ½ ozs. (16 crackers)	4 ozs. (24 crackers)
Muffins (English muffins, toasted)	70	4 ozs. (2 muffins)	6 ozs. (3 muffins)
Baked potato (without fat)	93	approx 12 ozs. (3 small)	approx 21 ozs. (5 small)
Rice, short grain	72	6 ozs. (1 heaping cup)	9 ⅔ ozs. (2 heaping cups)

Life Savers™	70	1 ¾ ozs. (2 packets)	2 ⅔ ozs. (3 packets)
Jelly beans	80	2 ozs. (25 jelly beans)	3 ozs. (38 jelly beans)
Watermelon	72	approx 32 ozs. (5 cups)	54 ozs. (7 ½ cups)
Sports electrolyte drink (6% carbohydrate)	73–78	28 ozs.	42 oz.

Females weighing about 110 lbs. should aim to eat 50 grams of carbohydrate. Males weighing about 165 lbs. should aim to eat 75 grams of carbohydrate.

RECOVERY FORMULA

Aim to ingest about 0.5 gram of carbohydrate per pound of body weight each 2 hours after exercise. If you weigh between 110 and 165 pounds, you need 55 to 80 grams of carbohydrate for each 2 hours after exercise.

If you want to keep up the pace from one training session to another, day after day, you will benefit by learning to select high G.I. foods. The trouble is that many people, even coaches and sports medicine practitioners, have got it all wrong when it comes to selecting sources of fast-release carbohydrate. The information in this chapter gives you the most up-to-date information and the key to better performance and faster recovery. Go for it!

HOW MUCH FOOD DO YOU NEED TO EAT TO GET THIS MUCH CARBOHYDRATE?

The table on page 86 gives the serving size of food and drinks containing 50 grams and 75 grams of carbohydrate. You need to choose a larger than normal serving. You may not feel like a meal of rice or pasta and this is the point where sports drinks and soft drinks on the market can help. Choose what you can tolerate and what is easy and practical for you to bring or buy. The main point is to make sure you eat and drink carbohydrate soon after the exercise session.

TO MAXIMIZE GLYCOGEN REPLENISHMENT AFTER THE COMPETITION

1. Ingest carbohydrate as soon as you can after the event and maintain a high carbohydrate intake for the next 24 hours.
2. Consume at least 5 grams of carbohydrate per pound of body weight over the 24 hours following prolonged exercise.
3. Choose high G.I. foods in the replenishment phase.
4. Avoid alcohol, which delays glycogen re-synthesis.

THE TRAINING DIET AND CARBOHYDRATE LOADING

It's not just your pre- and post-event meals that influence your performance. Consuming a high carbohydrate diet every day will help you reach peak performance. The glycemic index of the carbohydrate is not important here, only the amount of carbohydrate. It has been proven scientifically, unlike many other rumors involving dietary supplements, that eating lots of high carbohydrate foods will maximize muscle glycogen stores and thereby increase endurance.

The reason for this is that carbohydrate stores need to be replenished after each training session, not just after a race. If you train on a number of days per week, make sure you consume a high carbohydrate diet throughout the whole week.

Remember that alcohol interferes with glycogen re-synthesis and lowers blood glucose levels, sometimes to dangerous levels. Keep alcohol intake moderate—no more than one to three standard drinks per day and try to have two alcohol-free days a week. A standard drink is equivalent to one glass of wine (4-5 ounces), one can of beer (12 ounces) or one shot of distilled spirits (1.5 ounces).

BEER IS NOT A GOOD SOURCE OF CARBOHYDRATE.

When athletes fail to consume adequate carbohydrate each day, muscle and liver glycogen stores may eventually became depleted. Dr. Ted Costill at the University of Texas showed that the gradual and chronic depletion of stored glycogen may decrease endurance and exercise performance. Intense work-outs performed two to three times a day draw heavily on the athlete's muscle glycogen stores. Athletes on a low carbohydrate diet will not perform their best because muscle stores of fuel are low.

If the diet provides inadequate amounts of carbohydrate, the reduction in muscle glycogen will be critical. An athlete training heavily should consume about 500 to 800 grams of carbohydrate a day (about two to three times normal) to help prevent carbohydrate depletion. In practice, few athletes achieve this enormous figure. As a comparison, a typical man or woman eats only 240 grams of carbohydrate each day.

HOW DO YOU CHOOSE
A HIGH CARBOHYDRATE DIET?

The early chapters of this book provide all the practical tips you need for ensuring a high carbohydrate intake. In this chapter we give some extra pointers because very active people need to eat much larger amounts of carbohydrate than usual.

You may feel that you already know a lot about diet. But athletes, like everyone else, can have their facts wrong. Many foods that you believe are good sources of carbohydrate are even better sources of fat. For example, chocolate is 55 percent carbohydrate but also 30 percent fat. And fat won't help you win the race.

Dietary advice aimed at the general public needs to be modified for the serious athlete. Athletes have far greater energy needs, perhaps double that of the average office worker. Many high carbohydrate and low fat foods which are recommended for the average person are too bulky and satiating for athletes. It is their bulk that makes it difficult to consume the required amount of food. For example, a 75 gram carbohydrate portion of potatoes is equivalent to $1^1/_3$ pounds or 7 small potatoes—about four normal servings. Most people can't eat that much at a time. On the other hand, white bread is easy to eat in large amounts. A 75 gram carbohydrate portion of white bread is only five slices. Other foods that you might have believed were not so good for you, like soft drinks, candy, honey, sugar, flavored milk and ice cream are actually very concentrated sources of carbohydrate that can be used to supplement your diet.

Ian was manager of an under-18 men's hockey team. In addition to his role as manager, he was also in charge of the team's fitness and nutrition programs. He had done quite a lot of reading about the glycemic index and decided to base the whole diet around this.

Despite some early grumbling and moaning, the players stuck to the diet almost 100 percent during the whole two weeks of the championships. Ian planned the diet very carefully so that they got all the right foods at the right time—low G.I. before the game and high G.I. immediately after, along with jelly beans at half time.

He noticed that the benefits became very apparent early in the championship. The players themselves were noticing that they were not running out of energy during the game and were recovering a lot quicker than they had in the past.

About half way through the tournament other people started to wonder just where this team was getting all its energy.

"At first they thought it was amusing and perhaps a little strange that we were eating Cocoa Krispies and Rice Krispies at the team bus in the parking lot immediately after each game, but soon their amusement turned to curiosity," Ian said.

"People kept commenting on how fit the team was. But I knew that it wasn't just their fitness. I had not had as much time as I would have liked to work on their fitness, and in fact I remember being concerned just before we went away that their fitness levels may not have been high enough. I knew that what I was seeing was not just their fitness—it was the combination of fitness and a sustained energy supply. A 'whole body fitness' was what we had achieved. It clearly demonstrated to me that you cannot do one without the other.

"We ended up winning the championship by a relatively easy margin, and our fitness and energy levels were certainly a major contributing factor.

"One of the things I liked about using the glycemic index as the basis of the diet was that the players were able to very quickly understand the basic principles and by the end of the first week they knew exactly what to do.

"I gave the players a questionnaire to complete at the conclusion of the tournament, and I thought you would be interested to hear some of their comments."

- "I felt that when I played each game I was at my peak. I believe the diet played a major part in this."
- "I found I had more energy coming into and during the game."
- "Energy and glycogen levels were at perfect level."
- "I never felt flat or without energy."
- "Felt really good after every game, never felt run down during the game."
- "Everything made me feel good before, during and after the game."
- "Diet was major reason we did do well in the championships."
- "Feel better after games, recovery is better, better energy in the game."
- "I was never short of energy. My glycogen levels were constantly maintained and replenished at the necessary points. I always felt fit and healthy."
- "Kept my energy level high in the game and also after the game."
- "After the game, recovery is far more rapid."

IS YOUR DIET FIT FOR PEAK PERFORMANCE?

Take the diet fitness quiz and see how well you score. It's a good idea to use this quiz regularly to pick up on areas where you may need to improve your diet.

1. Circle your answer.

Eating patterns

- I eat at least 3 meals a day with no longer than 5 hours in between
  Yes/No

Carbohydrate checker

- I eat at least 4 slices of bread each day (1 roll = 2 slices of bread
  Yes/No
- I eat at least 1 cup of breakfast cereal each day or an extra slice of bread
  Yes/No
- I usually eat 2 or more pieces of fruit each day
  Yes/No
- I eat at least 3 different vegetables or have a salad most days
  Yes/No
- I include carbohydrates like pasta, rice and potato in my diet each day
  Yes/No

Protein checker

- I eat at least 1 and usually 2 servings of meat or meat alternatives (poultry, seafood, eggs, dried peas/beans or nuts) each day
  Yes/No

Fat checker

- I spread butter thinly on bread or use none at all
  Yes/No
- I eat fried food no more than once per week
  Yes/No
- I use polyunsaturated or monounsaturated oil (Canola or olive) for cooking. (Circle yes if you never fry in oil or fat)
  Yes/No
- I avoid oil-based dressings on salads
  Yes/No
- I use reduced fat or low fat dairy products
  Yes/No
- I cut the fat off meat and take the skin off chicken
  Yes/No
- I eat fatty snacks such as chocolate, potato chips, cookies or rich desserts/cakes etc. no more than twice a week
  Yes/No
- I eat fast or take-out food no more than once per week
  Yes/No

Iron checker

- I eat lean red meat at least 3 times per week or 2 servings of white meat daily or for vegetarians, include at least 1–2 cups of dried peas and beans (e.g. lentils, soy beans, chick peas) daily
  Yes/No
- I include a vitamin C source with meals based on bread, cereals, fruit and vegetables to assist the iron absorption in these "plant" sources of iron
  Yes/No

Calcium checker

- I eat at least 3 servings of dairy food or soy milk alternative each day (1 serving = 8 ounces milk or fortified soy milk; 1 slice (1 ounce) hard cheese; 8 ounces yogurt)
  Yes/No

Fluids

- I drink fluids regularly before, during and after exercise
  Yes/No

Alcohol

- When I drink alcohol, I would mostly drink no more than is recommended for the drunk driving limit
  Yes/No
  (Circle yes if you don't drink alcohol)

2. Score 1 point for every 'yes' answer

Scoring scale

18–20 Excellent   15–17 Room for improvement
12–14 Just made it   0–12 Poor

Note: Very active people will need to eat more breads, cereals and fruit than on this quiz, but to stay healthy no one should be eating less.

■ ■ ■

FURTHER READING ABOUT SPORTS NUTRITION

Williams M. Nutrition for Fitness and Sport, Fourth Edition. Brown & Benchmark, 1995

Berning J.R., Nelson Steen S. Nutrition for Sport & Exercise, Second Edition. Aspen, 1998

Clark N. Nancy Clark's Sports Nutrition Guidebook, Second Edition. Leisure Press, 1997

Chapter 7

THE GLYCEMIC INDEX AND DIABETES

The glycemic index has far-reaching implications for diabetes. Not only is it important in treating people with diabetes, but it may also help prevent people from getting diabetes in the first place and possibly even prevent some of the complications of diabetes.

WHAT IS DIABETES?

Diabetes is a chronic condition in which there is too much sugar (glucose) in the blood. Keeping the sugar level normal in the blood needs the right amount of a hormone called **insulin**. Insulin gets the sugar out of the blood and into the body's muscles where it is used to provide energy for the body. If there is not enough insulin or if the insulin does not do its job properly, diabetes develops.

In general, children and young adults develop diabetes because they cannot make enough insulin (type 1 diabetes). People over the age of 40 usually develop diabetes because their insulin does not work properly (type 2 diabetes). At first the body struggles to make extra insulin because what is there is not working properly, but later these people also develop a shortage of insulin. The aim of treatment for people with type 2 diabetes is to help them make the best use of the insulin they have and to try to make it last as long as possible.

Type 1, or insulin-dependent diabetes mellitus, occurs most commonly in children and young adults. In this type of diabetes the pancreas does not produce enough insulin and insulin injections are needed to replace the insulin deficit. Five percent of people with diabetes have type 1 diabetes; and,

Type 2, or non-insulin-dependent diabetes mellitus, typically occurs in older adults. These people are usually overweight and their insulin does not work properly. Medication or insulin injections may be necessary to treat this type of diabetes. Ninety percent of people with diabetes have type 2 diabetes.

Diabetes is on its way to becoming the most common health problem in the world. Currently, in many developing and newly industrialized nations, there is an epidemic of diabetes. Already in some countries half of the adult population has diabetes. In the United States, 16 million people have diabetes, about half of whom are not aware that they have the disease. It is the fourth-leading cause of death by disease, and the most prevalent chronic disease in children. Type 2 diabetes is more common among African-Americans, Hispanics, and Native Americans than in the general population.

WHY DO PEOPLE GET DIABETES?

The most common type of diabetes (type 2 diabetes) is the result of insulin not working properly and usually affects people over the age of 40. Overeating, being overweight and not exercising enough are important factors (what we call lifestyle factors) which can lead to this type of diabetes, especially when there is someone else in the family with diabetes.

Many people who live in societies which are undergoing rapid westernization are developing this type of diabetes. Why?

To find the answer we need to look back in time. Our ancestors lived and evolved in a very cold climate. Over the last 700,000 years there have been many ice ages—the last ended only 10,000 years ago. During these ice ages there was very little plant food around and people had to hunt and fish for survival. This gave them a lot of protein in their diet. In other words, during the ice ages our ancestors were carnivores (meat eaters). Their bodies adapted to this way of life to help them survive on this diet—and also to help them survive times when food was scarce.

As it turned out, this protein-based diet would also have protected them from developing diabetes. This is because the main way the body copes when there is not much carbohydrate (glucose) in the diet, is to make sure that the important parts, such as the brain, get what little glucose that is available. To do this the body makes very little insulin, because the brain can use glucose without insulin. Thus the body's demand for insulin was very small.

Since the end of the last ice age there have been many changes to the type and amount of food that we eat. First, our ancestors began to grow food crops. Agriculture changed their eating pattern from one based on protein to one based on carbohydrate in the form of whole cereal grains, vegetables and beans. A dietary change like this would also have changed the sugar levels in their blood. While they ate a high protein diet, the sugar levels in their blood would not have risen significantly after a meal. When they started eating carbohydrate regularly, the blood sugar level would have increased after meals. The amount by which the sugar levels in the blood increase after a meal depends on the glycemic index of the carbohydrate. Crops such as wheat grain, which our ancestors grew, have a low glycemic index. They would not have caused much change in blood sugar levels, so there would have been no need to use up much insulin, either.

The second major change came with industrialization and the advent of high speed steel roller mills. Instead of eating whole grain products, the new milling procedures broke up the grain into small particles, enabling us to produce flour so fine it resembled talcum powder. The end result was highly refined carbohydrate. We now know that breaking up natural grain seeds by milling leads to an increase in the glycemic index of a food, and transforms a low G.I. food into one with a high glycemic index. When this highly refined food is eaten it causes a greater increase in blood sugar levels. To keep the blood sugar levels normal, the body has to make large amounts of insulin. Many of the commercially packaged foods and drinks with which we now fill our shopping carts, have a high glycemic index. All this strains the body's insulin supplies.

Thirdly, the dramatic increase over the past 50 years in the quantity of high fat takeout and fast foods that we regularly eat has made matters even worse. So to our already high G.I. foods, we have added a lot of fat as well. As explained in Chapter 5, eating a lot of fat will increase body weight, which in turn makes it harder for the insulin to clear the glucose from the blood. In other words the body becomes insulin resistant—resistant to the effect of insulin. Continually eating carbohydrate foods with a high glycemic index places even more pressure on the body's ability to keep producing large amounts of insulin to control the blood sugar levels. Add to this insulin resistance, and you have the perfect recipe for eventually exhausting the body's insulin supply and developing diabetes. Recent studies from Harvard University's School of Public Health have shown that diets with low fiber and a high glycemic index increase the risk of developing type 2 diabetes by as much as two to three times. These studies, involving nearly 70,000 women and 50,000 men, controlled for factors that included body weight, smoking, total calorie intake and amount of carbohydrate. According to these researchers, the glycemic index of the diet is a much more important factor in promoting diabetes than the amount or type of fat.

It takes time for our bodies to adapt to such major changes in diet. Because our European ancestors had thousands of years to adapt to a diet with a lot of carbohydrate, they were in a better position to cope with the changes in the glycemic index of foods. That is why people of European extraction have a lower prevalence of type 2 diabetes compared with people whose diets have recently changed to include lots of high G.I. foods.

However, there is only so much that our bodies can take. As we continue to consume increasing quantities of foods with a high glycemic index plus excessive amounts of fatty foods, our bodies are coping less well. The result can be seen as a significant increase in the number of people developing diabetes.

But, the most dramatic increases in diabetes have occurred in populations which have been exposed to these changes over a very much shorter period of time. In some groups of Native Americans and in populations within the Oceania region, up to one adult in two has diabetes because of the rapid dietary and lifestyle changes in the twentieth century.

TREATING DIABETES

Taking care with what you eat is essential if you have diabetes. For some people with type 2 diabetes, this is all they have to do to keep their blood sugar levels in the normal range of between 70-140 mg/dL. Others also need to take pills or injections of insulin. People with type 1 diabetes must have insulin injections. But no matter what the treatment, everyone with diabetes must take care with what they eat in order to keep their blood sugar levels under control. Keeping the blood sugar near the normal range helps prevent complications of diabetes such as blindness, heart attacks, kidney failure and amputations.

For over a hundred years, people with diabetes have been given advice on what to eat. Many diets were based more on unproven (although seemingly logical) theories, rather than actual research. In 1915, for example, the *Boston Medical and Surgical Journal* advocated that the best dietary treatment for someone with diabetes was "limitation of all components of the diet." This translated into a very low calorie diet interspersed with days of fasting. Unfortunately, malnutrition was often the result.

In the 1920s doctors began recommending high fat diets for their patients. Ignorant of the dangers of a high fat diet, they knew that fat, at least, didn't break down to become blood sugar. We now know that high fat diets only hastened the development of heart disease, the most frequent cause of death among people with diabetes.

It was not until the 1970s that carbohydrate was considered to be a valuable part of the diabetic diet. Researchers found that not only did the nutritional status of patients improve with a higher carbohydrate intake, but their blood sugar levels improved as well.

The only part of food which directly affects blood sugar levels is carbohydrate. When we eat carbohydrate foods, they are broken down into sugar and cause the blood sugar levels to rise. The body responds by releasing insulin into the blood. The insulin clears the sugar from the blood, moving it into the muscles where it is used for energy, so the blood sugar level returns to normal.

Some people think that because carbohydrate raises the blood sugar level, it should not be eaten at all by people who have diabetes. This is not correct. Carbohydrate is a normal part of the diet and at least half of our total daily calories should come from carbohydrate. In fact, the more carbohydrate you eat the better, because it automatically reduces the proportion of calories you get from fat.

THE SECRET TO THE DIABETIC DIET

IS NOT ONLY THE QUANTITY BUT ALSO

THE TYPE OF CARBOHYDRATE.

Traditionally sugar was excluded from diabetic diets because it was thought to be the worst type of carbohydrate. The simple structure of sugar supposedly made it more rapidly digested and absorbed than other types of carbohydrate, like starch. This assumption was simply not correct. Even in the late 1970s, test meal studies showed that there was a great deal of overlap between the blood sugar responses to sugary and starchy foods. Fifty grams of carbohydrate eaten as potato caused a higher rise in blood sugar than 50 grams of sugar. Ice cream resulted in a lower blood sugar response than potato! Findings like these sparked research into the glycemic index in an effort to learn more about how the body actually responds to different carbohydrate foods.

In the United States, the emphasis has been on the quantity of carbohydrate in the diet. "Portion" diets or "exchanges" are used to prescribe a set amount of carbohydrate to be eaten at every meal. (A "carbohydrate portion" is an amount of carbohydrate-rich food which contains 15 grams of carbohydrate.)

An underlying assumption of the carbohydrate portions theory is that equivalent **amounts** of carbohydrate, regardless of the **type**, cause an equal change in the blood sugar level. The American Diabetes Association (ADA) continues to press this line of thinking and no longer makes a distinction between even starch and sugars. But unfortunately, the ADA has not recognized that differences in blood sugar responses among foods—the glycemic index of foods—are large enough to warrant any change to the current system of carbohydrate counting. In truth, there are more published studies supporting the usefulness of the glycemic index approach in diabetes control than there are of carbohydrate portions. The authors of this book, along with other experts, believe that both the *amount* and *type* of carbohydrate must be considered. In Canada, Europe, Australia and New Zealand, the diabetes and dietetic associations have recommended that low glycemic index foods be emphasized in the dietary management of diabetes.

The glycemic index has shown us that the way to increase the quantity of carbohydrate in the diabetic diet, without increasing the sugar levels in the blood, is to choose carbohydrate foods with a low glycemic index.

At 50 years of age, Helen had tried many times to lose weight. Her neighbors had started walking on a regular basis but she felt tired all the time and had no energy to do anything more than what she had to. Being 209 pounds and only 5 feet, 5 ½ inches tall ruined her morale. Her mother had diabetes and she knew being overweight put her at greater risk, but every time she lost weight she ended up regaining it. Finally, it was no surprise to her when she was diagnosed with diabetes. In fact it was some relief, here at last was a reason for her tiredness.

On her doctor's suggestion, Helen saw a dietitian for help with her diet. At first glance what Helen was eating appeared reasonable. Breakfast was a slice of whole wheat toast or a whole wheat cracker with butter and black tea. Lunch was a light meal such as celery, lettuce, a slice of cheese, a slice of cold meat, an egg and a couple of crackers, spread with butter. For dinner she was having soup and a piece of steak with vegetables. She limited herself to a small cocktail potato. The meal was finished by a piece of fruit.

A closer look at her food record, showed that Helen's diet was in fact poorly balanced. It was dominated by protein and fat foods and contained insufficient carbohydrate. It didn't contain enough food to provide a good range of nutrients. What's more, Helen herself was struggling with it and often felt hungry since she had cut candy and cookies out of her diet.

To improve things, we first looked at the frequency of eating. Helen kept to three meals a day because she had been brought up to believe that was better for her. She agreed to trying a small snack of fruit or a slice of bread between meals. Even though she wasn't on medication for diabetes, the effect of spreading her food intake more evenly across the day, between small meals and snacks, could help to stabilize her blood sugar level and help her lose weight.

We then revised the amount of carbohydrate that she ate, and listed a range of low G.I. carbohydrate foods that were to be her **first priority** at each meal. The filling value of the carbohydrate left her with less space for the proteins that used to dominate her diet. Helen's new diet looked more like this:

Breakfast began with a fresh orange, juiced, and a bowl of oats with raisins and 1% milk. Helen added a slice of whole grain bread or raisin toast if she was still hungry.

Lunch was usually a sandwich on 100% stoneground whole wheat bread with a slice of lean meat and salad and a piece of fruit to finish. Sometimes she had a vegetable soup or pasta with a vegetable sauce and salad.

The proportion of foods on her **dinner** plate was rearranged, shrinking in the meat department and filling out on the vegetable side. She began to think of carbohydrate food as the basis of the meal and varied between pasta, rice and potato. Twice a week she made a vegetarian dish with legumes like a minestrone soup or a vegetable lasagna. An evening snack was usually yogurt or fruit.

After a month on her new eating plan Helen felt better—in fact she felt well enough to tackle some exercise. Taking a serious look at her day, she decided to commit the half hour after dinner to a walk, five nights a week.

Over the next six months Helen's weight dropped from 200 pounds to 175 pounds. Her blood sugar levels were mainly within the normal range. She no longer struggled with hunger and felt good about the food she was eating.

Lowering the glycemic index of your diet as Helen did is not as hard as it seems, because just about every carbohydrate food that you eat has an equivalent food with a low glycemic index. Our research has shown that blood sugar levels in people with diabetes are greatly improved if foods with a low glycemic index are substituted for high glycemic index foods.

We studied a group of people with diabetes and taught them how to alter their diet by substituting the high G.I. foods they were normally eating for carbohydrate foods with a low glycemic index. After three months, there was a significant fall in their blood sugar levels. They did not find the diet at all difficult and in fact commented on how easy it had been to make the change and how much more variety had been introduced to their diet.

Bill, a 62-year-old man, was taking every care with his diabetes. He had changed his diet by reducing his total food intake, had lost weight and was exercising regularly. He was testing his blood sugar levels at home. Despite his best efforts, he could not achieve a blood sugar level in the desired range of below 140 mg/dL after breakfast. At first glance he was eating what most dietitians would consider to be a good breakfast for someone with diabetes: 1 cup of cornflakes with 8 ounces of milk plus 2 slices of whole wheat toast with a little margarine. However, his blood sugar after breakfast was consistently around 200 mg/dL. He was advised to make one simple change—to lower the glycemic index of the carbohydrate by changing the corn flakes to a bowl of rolled oats. This had an immediate impact and his sugar levels after breakfast fell to 126 mg/dL.

SUBSTITUTING LOW G.I. FOODS FOR HIGH G.I. FOODS—WHAT TO CHANGE

High G.I. Food	Low G.I. Alternative
Bread, whole wheat or white	Bread containing a lot of whole grains, sourdough bread, 100% stoneground whole wheat bread, whole grain pumpernickel
Many highly processed breakfast cereals	Unrefined cereal such as oats, or check the G.I. list for processed cereals with a low glycemic index (e.g. All Bran™
Plain cookies and crackers	Cookies made with dried fruit and whole grains such as oats
Cakes and muffins	Look for those made with fruit, oats, whole grains
Tropical fruits such as bananas	Temperate climate fruits such as apples, peaches, nectarines, etc.
Potato	Substitute occasionally with pasta or legumes
Rice	Try Basmati or Uncle Ben's Converted™ Rice

Check the G.I. list at the back of the book for many more low G.I. alternatives.

So, making this type of change in the everyday diet does not mean that the diet has to be restrictive or impossible to eat. Many recipes in this book can help you reduce the glycemic index of your diet. The following case history is an example of the results you could obtain. If you are having trouble controlling your blood sugar level after a meal look up the glycemic index for the carbohydrates it contains. See if you can find substitutes with a lower glycemic index among the list. Eating a meal with a lower glycemic index can lower the blood sugar rise after the meal.

Although we haven't mentioned them yet, don't think that fatty foods are not important. They are, especially in people who are overweight. But fatty foods do not increase blood sugar levels. Only carbohydrate foods do. However, being overweight and eating fatty foods **prevents** the body's insulin from doing its job and indirectly causes the blood sugar levels to rise. So, eating French fries, a mixtures of high G.I. carbohydrate and fat, causes double trouble. Not only does the high glycemic index of potato increase the blood sugar levels, but the extra fat will also eventually stop the body's insulin from working properly and makes it less effective in clearing the sugar from the blood. Persistently high blood sugar levels will ultimately damage the body.

The glycemic index is especially important when carbohydrate is eaten by itself and not as part of a mixed meal. Carbohydrate tends to have a stronger effect on our blood sugar level when it is eaten alone. This is the case with between-meal snacks which most people with diabetes have to have. When choosing a between-meal snack, pick one with a low glycemic index. For example, an apple with a glycemic index of 36 is better than a slice of normal toast with a glycemic index of around 70, and will result in less of a jump in the blood sugar level.

A NOTE OF CAUTION

Some snack foods with a very low glycemic index (such as peanuts, which have a glycemic index of 14) have a very high fat content and are not recommended for people with a weight problem. As an occasional snack they are fine (especially as their fat is monounsaturated), but not every day. Peanuts are also very tempting, and it is hard to stop at just one handful!

LOW FAT AND LOW G.I. SNACK FOODS

Stoneground whole wheat raisin-bread toast
Low fat milkshake or smoothie
An apple
Low fat fruit yogurt

Dried apricots
Peaches and plums
Baked beans
An orange
Popcorn
A glass of 1% milk

Leanne was seven and a half months pregnant when she developed gestational diabetes. Her doctor advised her to keep her blood sugar level after meals less than 126 mg/dL. To check this, Leanne performed finger-prick blood tests on herself every day. The only time she found her blood sugar tended to be higher than 126 mg/dL was after her main meal in the evening. By looking back over the results of her home blood sugar monitoring, she found that her blood sugar was high if she ate potato but fine when she had pasta. The secret to good blood sugars for Leanne? Pasta more often, and inclusion of low G.I. carbohydrate whenever she had potato.

Many people with diabetes have to resort to pills to control blood sugar levels. The following story shows you how an increased intake of low G.I. carbohydrate foods can sometimes make pills unnecessary.

Mary, 65 years old, was found to have diabetes two years ago. She was overweight and was told that she had to lose several pounds. Although she had been trying to do this before she developed diabetes, she had been unsuccessful. Now she felt that the extra burden of diabetes would make life impossible for her and that she could not do any more than she was already doing with her diet. Because her blood sugar levels were too high, she was given diabetic medication.

When we looked at what Mary ate, we could see that indeed she really was trying hard and was not overeating. However, almost all of her carbohydrate foods had a high glycemic index. For example, she was having shredded wheat or cornflakes for breakfast, crackers for mid-meal snacks, bread with her lunch and evening meals and watermelon was a favorite fruit.

All these foods have a high glycemic index. By changing to All-Bran or untoasted muesli for breakfast, having oatmeal cookies or an apple, pear or orange for snacks and by adjusting the type and amount of bread she was eating, Mary was able to eat more, lose weight and improve her blood sugar levels. Eventually she stopped having to take her diabetes pills, too.

Sometimes, despite your best efforts with diet, medication will still be needed to obtain good blood sugar control. This is eventually the case for most people with type 2 diabetes.

HYPOGLYCEMIA—THE EXCEPTION TO THE LOW G.I. RULE

In people with diabetes who are treated with insulin or medication, the blood sugar may sometimes fall below 70 mg/dL which is the lower end of the normal range. When this happens you might feel hungry, shaky and sweaty, and be unable to think clearly. This is called a reaction (short for hypoglycemic reaction).

A reaction is a potentially dangerous situation and must be treated immediately by eating some carbohydrate food. In this case you should pick a carbohydrate with a high glycemic index because you need to increase your blood sugar quickly. Glucose tablets, which are widely available and which many diabetics keep with them for these low blood-sugar moments, are a great source of instant carbohydrate. Jelly beans (with a glycemic index of 80) or dried dates (with a G.I. of 103) are other good choices. If you are not due for your next meal or snack you should also have some low G.I. carbohydrate, like an apple, to keep your blood sugar from falling again until you next eat.

Reactions in the night were a particularly worrying problem for Jane. Her evening insulin doses had been adjusted in an effort to stop her blood sugar levels from falling too low at night, but she believed experimenting with her supper carbohydrate could also help. After trying many different foods and frequently testing her blood-sugar levels at 3 am, she discovered an answer that the glycemic index predicted would work—milk! Jane found that a large glass of milk before going to bed, rather than her usual plain cookies was easy to have, and maintained her blood sugar at a good level through the night.

DIABETES COMPLICATIONS

If blood sugar levels are not properly controlled, diabetes can cause damage to the blood vessels in the heart, legs, brain, eyes and kidneys. For this reason, heart attacks, leg amputations, strokes, blindness and kidney failure are more common in people with diabetes. It can also damage the nerves in the feet causing pain and irritation in the feet and numbness and loss of sensation.

Many researchers believe that high levels of insulin also contribute to the damage of the blood vessels of the heart, legs and brain. High insulin levels are thought to be one of the factors which might stimulate the muscle in the wall of the blood vessel to thicken. Thickening of the muscle wall causes the blood vessels to narrow and can slow the flow of blood to the point that a clot can form and stop the blood flow altogether. This is what happens to cause a heart attack or stroke.

We know that foods with a high glycemic index cause the body to produce larger amounts of insulin, resulting in higher levels of insulin in the blood. Therefore, for people with type 2 diabetes, it makes sense that eating foods with a low glycemic index will have the effect of helping to control blood sugar levels, and will do this with lower levels of insulin. This may have the added benefit of reducing the large vessel damage which accounts for so many of the problems of diabetes.

PREVENTING TYPE 2 DIABETES

Most people who develop type 2 diabetes have a tendency to be unable to produce enough insulin to control their blood sugar levels. Remember, high G.I. foods increase the amount of insulin the body needs, so, for those people susceptible to diabetes, eating carbohydrate with a high glycemic index will only increase the demand on their already struggling pancreas.

Who is likely to be at risk? People who are over the age of 50, have a family history of diabetes, are overweight, have high blood pressure or have had diabetes during pregnancy (gestational diabetes) are at risk of developing type 2 diabetes. A reduction of the glycemic index of their diet reduces the demand on their pancreas to produce more insulin, perhaps prolonging its function and delaying the development of diabetes.

If you fit into one of these categories, you can reduce your chances of getting diabetes by controlling your weight, exercising more and eating more foods with a low glycemic index.

SYNDROME X

Over the past ten years it has become apparent that a number of health problems which cause heart attacks are found together in many people. These include high blood sugar levels, high blood fat levels (especially triglycerides), obesity, high blood pressure and increased blood clotting. When these are found together they are referred to as Syndrome X.

The underlying problems in people with Syndrome X are that the body is insensitive to insulin and there are high levels of insulin in the blood. These high insulin levels are thought to cause many of the problems found in this syndrome. There are a number of ways that high insulin levels can cause high blood pressure.

High insulin levels in the blood after eating are the result of the carbohydrate in the food. As we have shown before, the high glycemic index foods cause much higher insulin levels than low glycemic index foods. One way of controlling the high insulin levels in the blood is to eat low glycemic index foods. Such a diet will help correct many of the problems found in Syndrome X.

A WORD OF ADVICE

There are many factors that can affect your blood sugar levels. If you have diabetes and you are struggling to control your blood sugar level it is important to seek medical help. How much exercise you do, your weight, stress levels, total dietary intake and need for medication may have to be assessed.

ODE TO THE GLYCEMIC INDEX
by Martina Chippindall

Mirror, mirror on the wall
What's the fastest of them all?
Sugars, starches, grains or grapes
Please tell me how to fill my plate!

For years I followed all the rules
And was often made to feel a fool
When no explanation could be found
Why my sugars were always up and down

At last research has laid to rest
The myth that sugar's not the best.
In fact an index has been found
Which gives us greater choice, all round!

Chapter 8

THE GLYCEMIC INDEX AND HYPOGLYCEMIA

TREATING HYPOGLYCEMIA

*H*ypoglycemia is a condition in which the sugar level in the blood falls below normal levels. From the Greek words *hypo* meaning under and *glycemia* meaning blood sugar—hence blood sugar level below normal.

These days, hypoglycemia is a popular diagnosis for all sorts of problems which cannot be attributed to a more specific diagnosis. There has been considerable publicity about hypoglycemia which is often blamed for many non-specific health problems ranging from tiredness to depression. Unfortunately, it is often wrongly blamed, which can delay a proper diagnosis and correct treatment.

Nevertheless, genuine hypoglycemia does occur in a few people, and the glycemic index has a role to play in treating some forms of this condition. The most common form of hypoglycemia occurs after a meal is eaten. This is called **reactive hypoglycemia**.

Normally, when a meal containing carbohydrate is eaten, the

blood sugar level rises. This causes the pancreas to make insulin which "pushes" the sugar out of the blood and into the muscles where it provides energy for you to carry out your regular tasks and activities. The movement of sugar out of the blood and into the muscles is finely controlled by just the right amount of insulin to drop the sugar back to normal. In some people, the blood sugar level rises too quickly after eating and causes an **excessive** amount of insulin to be released. This draws too much sugar out of the blood and causes the blood sugar level to fall below normal. The result is hypoglycemia.

Hypoglycemia causes a variety of unpleasant symptoms. Many of these are stress-like symptoms such as sweating, tremor, anxiety, palpitations and weakness. Others affect mental function and lead to restlessness, irritability, poor concentration, lethargy and drowsiness.

The diagnosis of true reactive hypoglycemia cannot be made on the basis of vague symptoms. It depends on detecting a low blood sugar level when the symptoms are actually being experienced. This means a blood test.

Because it may be difficult (or almost impossible) for someone to be in the right place at the right time to have a blood sample taken while experiencing the symptoms, a glucose tolerance test is sometimes used to try to make the diagnosis. This involves drinking pure glucose, which causes the blood sugar levels to rise. If too much insulin is produced in response, a person with reactive hypoglycemia will experience an excessive fall in their blood sugar level. It sounds simple enough, but there are pitfalls. Testing must be done under strictly controlled conditions and capillary (not venous) blood samples collected correctly. Home blood glucose meters are not sufficient for the diagnosis of hypoglycemia in people without diabetes.

TREATING HYPOGLYCEMIA

The aim of treating reactive hypoglycemia is to prevent sudden large increases in blood sugar levels. If the blood sugar level can be prevented from increasing quickly, then excessive unnecessary amounts of insulin will not be produced and the blood sugar levels will not plunge to abnormally low levels.

Smooth steady blood sugar levels can be readily achieved by changing from high to low G.I. foods in the diet. This is particularly important when eating carbohydrate foods by themselves. Low G.I. foods like whole grain bread, low fat yogurt and low G.I. fruits are best for snacks.

If you can stop the big swings in blood glucose levels, then you will not get the symptoms of reactive hypoglycemia and chances are you will feel a lot better.

Hypoglycemia due to a serious medical problem is rare. Such conditions require in-depth investigation and treatment of the underlying cause.

An irregular eating pattern is the most common dietary habit that we see in people who have hypoglycemia. The following case study illustrates this very well.

Diane, with her hectic working life, often did not find time for proper meals. Finally, her body no longer accepted the strain it was under. Diane began to experience odd bouts of weakness and shakiness where she was unable to think clearly. A visit to the doctor and a glucose tolerance test confirmed that she was suffering from hypoglycemia. The treatment was to change her habits—her eating pattern at least. Diane needed to eat three regular meals a day with snacks in between. The thought of eating six times every day seemed an enormous task to Diane—and it took much thought and planning to organize her new diet. What kept her going was how much better she felt almost immediately. The following meal plan is a typical menu for Diane's day.

Breakfast
6 AM
Banana, milk, yogurt, honey and vanilla blended into a smoothie for a speedy start to the day

At work
8.30 AM
An oatbran and apple muffin (homemade on the weekend and frozen individually)

Lunch
12 NOON
(New habit—must have every day)
A substantial sandwich, prepared with a low G.I. bread. Occasionally a Mexican dish with beans or pasta if eating out.

At work   Handful of dried apricots or apples (kept in jar in office)
3 PM

Still at work   Couple of oatmeal cookies (kept in office) for late days
5 PM

Dinner   Something quick, e.g. pasta, a baked-bean main
7.30 PM   dish, or meat and vegetables. (Always
double check for carbohydrate in the main course.)

Fruit or milkshake for dessert or late night snack

TO PREVENT HYPOGLYCEMIA, REMEMBER

- Eat regular meals and snacks—plan to eat every three hours or so
- Include low G.I. carbohydrate foods at every meal and for snacks
- Mix high G.I. foods with low G.I. foods in your meals—the combination will give an overall intermediate G.I.
- Avoid eating high G.I. foods on their own for snacks—this can trigger hypoglycemia

Chapter 9

THE GLYCEMIC INDEX AND HEART DISEASE

WHAT IS HEART DISEASE

WHY DO PEOPLE GET HEART DISEASE

RISK FACTORS FOR HEART DISEASE

TREATING HEART DISEASE: SECONDARY PREVENTION

PREVENTING HEART DISEASE: PRIMARY PREVENTION

THE GLYCEMIC INDEX AND HEART DISEASE

THE GLYCEMIC INDEX AND INSULIN SENSITIVITY

This chapter was originally written for the U.K. edition of this book by Dr. Anthony Leeds. As with the entirety of this book, it has been adapted for this edition. Dr. Leeds is Senior Lecturer in the Department of Nutrition at the University of London. He graduated in medicine from the Middlesex Hospital Medical School in 1971. He conducts research on carbohydrate and dietary fiber and their relation to high blood cholesterol, obesity and diabetes. He chairs the Forum on Food and Health at the Royal Society of Medicine and the Research Ethics Committee of King's College London.

The glycemic index is important in heart disease, too. It has a role in the diets of people who already have heart disease, but perhaps of greater significance in the long term, it has a practical role in the prevention of heart disease.

WHAT IS HEART DISEASE?

Most heart disease in the Western world, and increasingly elsewhere, is caused by atherosclerosis of the arteries, sometimes referred to as "hardening of the arteries." Most people develop atherosclerosis gradually during their lifetime. If it develops sufficiently slowly it may not cause any problems, even into great old age, but if its development is accelerated by one or more of many processes the condition may cause trouble much earlier in life.

Atherosclerosis results in reduced blood flow through the affected arteries. In the heart this can mean that the heart muscle gets insufficient oxygen to provide the power for pumping blood, and it changes in such a way that pain is experienced (central chest pain or angina pectoris). Elsewhere in the body, atherosclerosis has a similar blood flow reducing effect: in the legs it can cause muscle pains on exercise (intermittent claudication); in the brain it can cause a variety of problems from "funny turns" to strokes.

An even more serious consequence of atherosclerosis occurs when a blood clot forms over the surface of a patch of atherosclerosis on an artery. This process of thrombosis can result in a complete blockage of the artery with consequences ranging from sudden death to a small heart attack from which the patient recovers quickly. The process of thrombosis can occur elsewhere in the arterial system with a range of consequences determined by the extent of the thrombosis. The probability of developing thrombosis is determined by the "tendency" of the blood to clot versus the natural ability of the blood to break down clots (fibrinolysis). These two counteracting "tendencies" are influenced by a number of factors, including some dietary factors (most notably the effect of fatty fish or fish oils in the diet).

People who have gradually developed atherosclerosis of the arteries to the heart (the coronary arteries) may gradually develop reduced heart function. For a while the heart may be able to compensate for the problem, so there may be no symptoms, but eventually it may begin to fail. Shortness of breath may begin to occur, initially on exercise, and there may sometimes be some swelling of the ankles. Modern medicine has many effective drug treatments for heart failure so this consequence of atherosclerosis does not have quite the same serious implications as it did in the past.

WHY DO PEOPLE GET HEART DISEASE?

Atherosclerotic heart disease develops early in life when the many factors that cause it have a strong influence. Over many decades doctors and scientists have identified the processes in fine detail and now most of the factors which cause heart disease are well known. Theoretically this type of heart disease might be largely prevented if everyone's risks were assessed in youth and if all the right things were done throughout the rest of their lives. In practice there has been only a limited development of the ways to screen people for risk early in life, and the resources needed to achieve prevention are just not available. However a great deal is already being done to identify risk factors in healthy people and those with established heart disease. Those who take the necessary action reduce their risk.

RISK FACTORS FOR HEART DISEASE

The chance of developing heart disease is increased if you smoke tobacco, have high blood pressure, have diabetes, have high blood cholesterol (which may be due to eating too much fat in your diet), are overweight or obese and/or do not do enough physical exercise.

- Smoking of tobacco is now clearly established as a cause of atherosclerosis. Few authorities now dispute the evidence. There are however some interesting dietary aspects: Did you know that smokers tend to eat less fruit and vegetables compared to non-smokers (and thus eat less of the protective anti-oxidant plant compounds)? Did you know that smokers tend to eat more fat and more salt than non-smokers? These characteristics of the smoker's diet may be caused by a desire to seek stronger food flavors as a consequence of the taste-blunting effect of smoking. While these dietary differences may make the smoker at greater risk of heart disease there is only one piece of advice for anyone who smokes: **please stop smoking!**

■ High blood pressure causes changes in the walls of arteries. The muscle layer (remember an artery is not a rigid pipe, it is a muscular tube, which when healthy can change its size to control the flow of blood) becomes thickened and atherosclerosis is more likely to develop. Treatments for blood pressure have become more effective over the last thirty years, but it is only now becoming clear which types of treatment for blood pressure are also effective at reducing heart disease risk.

■ Diabetes is caused by a lack of insulin—either the body does not produce enough or the body "demands" more than normal (because it has become insensitive to insulin). In diabetes some of the chemical (metabolic) processes which take place tend to accelerate atherosclerosis. Diabetes may also result in raised blood fats. The increased risk of heart disease is a major reason why so much effort is put into achieving normal control of blood sugar in diabetic patients, and also why all people with diabetes should be checked for the other risk factors of heart disease.

■ High blood cholesterol increases the risk of heart disease. Your blood cholesterol is determined by genetic (inherited) factors—which you cannot change—and lifestyle factors—which you **can** change. There are some relatively rare conditions in which particularly high blood cholesterol levels occur. People who have inherited these conditions need a thorough "work-up" by a specialist doctor followed by life-long drug treatment. In most people high blood cholesterol is partly determined by their genes, which have "set" the cholesterol slightly high, and lifestyle factors which push it up more. The most important dietary factor is fat. The diets prescribed for blood cholesterol lowering are low fat (low saturated fat), high carbohydrate, high fiber diets. Body weight also affects blood cholesterol—in some people being overweight has a significant effect on the levels—attaining a reasonable weight can be helpful. The blood also contains triglycerides, another type of fat which is particularly high after meals. High triglycerides may be linked with increased risk of heart disease in some people.

■ Overweight and obese people are more likely to have high blood pressure and to have diabetes. They are also at increased risk of getting heart disease. Some of that increased risk is due to the high blood pressure, and the tendency to diabetes, but there is a separate "independent" effect of the obesity. When increased fatness develops it can be distributed evenly all over the body or it may occur centrally—in and around the abdomen (stomach). This central obesity is particularly strongly associated with the risk of heart disease. Thus every effort should be made to get body weights nearer to normal—especially if the extra weight is "middle-age spread."

■ Exercise has several benefits for the heart. Cardiovascular fitness is improved by regular strenuous exercise and the blood supply to the heart may be "improved." Exercise is also important in maintaining body weight and has effects on metabolism and some factors related to blood clotting. Getting regular exercise is clearly important.

TREATING HEART DISEASE: SECONDARY PREVENTION

When heart disease is detected two types of treatment are given. Firstly the effects of the disease are treated (e.g. medical treatment with drugs and surgical treatment to bypass blocked arteries) and, secondly, the risk factors are treated to slow down the further progression of the disease. Treatment of risk factors after the disease has already developed is "secondary prevention." In people who have not yet developed the disease, treatment of risk factors is "primary prevention." Obviously it would be better to give primary preventive treatment in all cases.

PREVENTING HEART DISEASE:
PRIMARY PREVENTION

More and more people now get regular checks of their blood pressure, and tests to check for diabetes. Increasingly blood fat tests are done to check this risk factor too. All health professionals give lifestyle advice on stopping smoking, the benefits of exercise and the nature of a good diet. When specific risk factors are discovered, diet and lifestyle advice is given, but sometimes may not be followed for long. It is especially difficult to follow advice if the effect of not following it is likely not to matter for ten or more years, and if the changes needed are not attractive. The changes must be wanted by the individual who will be helped by encouragement from friends and relatives, and the changes must ideally be positive changes—"I want to do this" not "They've told me to do this." Any new dimension in heart disease prevention must be seen as a great positive change rather than as negative.

THE GLYCEMIC INDEX AND HEART DISEASE

The glycemic index is highly relevant to prevention of heart disease. Since it has benefits for the overweight and those who have diabetes, a low G.I. diet may reduce the risk of heart disease by helping to reduce body weight and improve blood glucose control. In the Harvard Nurses' Study, those who ate a low G.I. diet had *half* the risk of actual heart attack compared to those on the highest G.I. diet.

Low G.I. diets also tend to reduce total blood cholesterol and low-density (LDL) cholesterol in some people (lower levels of total cholesterol and LDL cholesterol are associated with lower risk of heart disease. Sometimes this may be due to the fact that the low G.I. diet is usually low in fat and often a little lower in total energy (calorie) content, though there may be a direct effect of "low G.I." on blood cholesterol. Interestingly, in addition to these effects, low G.I. diets may influence the "good" cholesterol in blood, that is, the high-density (HDL) cholesterol. HDL cholesterol is a sign of cholesterol being taken away from arteries, so the higher the better. A study of the diets of over 1,400 middle-aged adults in Britain showed that the glycemic index of the diet was the only dietary variable significantly related to HDL cholesterol. People who had a low G.I. diet had high HDL cholesterol. Large-scale surveys have shown that high HDL cholesterol is associated with a lower risk of heart disease. This effect of the low G.I. diet may be due to the way such diets affect the body's sensitivity to insulin (see below) which in turn increases levels of HDL cholesterol.

THE GLYCEMIC INDEX AND INSULIN SENSITIVITY

At the end of Chapter 7 we referred to Syndrome X, a condition characterized by high blood sugar levels, high blood fat levels (especially triglycerides), obesity, high blood pressure and increased clotting, all associated with high blood insulin levels. However there is more to Syndrome X than this—in this condition it is now known that the body is insensitive to insulin. The tissues of the body change so that more insulin is needed to achieve the same effect as usual, and the body reponds by circulating more insulin in the blood. Tests on patients with heart disease show that a much higher than expected number of them have this insensitivity to insulin.

Can a low G.I. diet help? In a recent study, patients with serious disease of the coronary arteries were given either low or high G.I. diets before surgery for coronary bypass grafts. They were given blood tests before their diets and just before surgery, and at surgery small pieces of fat tissue were removed for testing. The tests on the fat showed that the low G.I. diets made the tissues of these "insulin insensitive" patients more sensitive—in fact they were back in the same range as normal "control" patients after just a few weeks on the diet.

If people with serious heart disease can be improved would the same happen with younger people? Young women in their thirties were divided into those who did and those who did not have a family history of heart disease. They themselves had not yet developed the condition. They had blood tests followed by low or high G.I. diets for four weeks, after which they had more blood tests, and then when they had surgery (for conditions unrelated to heart disease) pieces of fat were again removed and tested for insulin sensitivity. The young women with a family history of heart disease were insensitive to insulin (those without the family history of heart disease were normal) but after four weeks on the low G.I. diet were normal again.

In both studies the diets were designed to try to ensure that all the other variables (like total energy, total carbohydrates) were not different, so that the change in insulin sensitivity seen was likely to have been due to the low G.I. diet rather than any other factor.

Work on these exciting findings continues but what is known so far strongly suggests that low G.I. diets not only improve body weight and improve blood sugar in people with diabetes, but also improve the sensitivity of the body to insulin. It will take many years of further research to show that this simple dietary change to a low G.I. diet will definitely slow the progress of atherosclerotic heart disease. In the meantime it is clear that risk factors for heart disease are improved by the low G.I. diet. Low G.I. diets are consistent with the other required dietary changes needed for prevention of heart disease. So the message for heart disease prevention is: low fat (low saturated fat), high carbohydrate, high fiber, **low G.I.!**

THE MESSAGE FOR HEART DISEASE PREVENTION

IS LOW FAT (LOW SATURATED FAT),

HIGH CARBOHYDRATE, HIGH FIBER AND LOW G.I.

Part 2

YOUR GUIDE TO LOW G.I. EATING

MAKING THE CHANGE TO A LOW G.I. DIET

COOKING THE LOW G.I. WAY

THE RECIPES

■

Chapter 10

MAKING THE CHANGE TO A LOW G.I. DIET

CREATING MEALS TO ACHIEVE THE
GLYCEMIC INDEX YOU NEED

MAKING THE CHANGE TO A LOW G.I. DIET

BREAKFAST: USING THE GLYCEMIC INDEX TO
SUSTAIN YOU THROUGH THE DAY

A SIMPLE, HEALTHY LOW G.I. BREAKFAST

TEN QUICK LOW-FAT, LOW G.I. BREAKFAST IDEAS

LUNCH: IDEAS FOR A LIGHT MEAL
OR A G.I. LOWERING SIDE DISH

LUNCHING OUT

TEN LOW G.I. LUNCHES ON THE GO

MAIN MEALS: CHOOSING THE BEST WITH LOW G.I.

TEN LOW G.I. MAIN MEALS IN MINUTES

DESSERTS: A LOW G.I. FINISH

EIGHT QUICK AND EASY LOW G.I. DESSERTS

SNACKS: KEEPING YOUR ENERGY LEVELS UP
BETWEEN MEALS

SUSTAINING SNACKS

CREATING MEALS TO ACHIEVE
THE GLYCEMIC INDEX YOU NEED

Eating a low G.I. diet still means eating a variety of foods. Possibly a wider variety than you are already eating. Potatoes with a high G.I. can still be included. A food is not good or bad on the basis of its glycemic index. The glycemic index of a meal consisting of a mixture of carbohydrate foods is a weighted average of the G.I.s of the carbohydrate foods. The weighting is based on the proportion of the total carbohydrate contributed by each food. Usually we eat a combination of carbohydrate foods, sandwiches and fruit, pasta and bread, baked beans with a hot dog on a bun, cereal and toast, potatoes and corn. Studies show that when a food with a high glycemic index is combined with a food with a low glycemic index, the complete meal has an intermediate glycemic index.

HIGH GLYCEMIC INDEX FOOD + LOW GLYCEMIC INDEX FOOD =

INTERMEDIATE GLYCEMIC INDEX MEAL

Supposing you have a meal of baked beans with a hot dog and bun.

Regular white bread has a glycemic index of 70, and baked beans have a glycemic index of 48.

If we assume half the carbohydrate is coming from the bread, and half from the baked beans, we can add the glycemic index values of the two foods together and divide by 2: (70 + 48) ÷ 2. This gives the meal a final glycemic index of 59.

The final glycemic index of a meal depends on the glycemic index values of the foods that make up the meal and the proportion of carbohydrate contributed by each carbohydrate rich food.

If you have two carbohydrate rich foods combined 50:50, you can add their G.I. values and halve the result to come up with the new glycemic index. But if you have two foods combined in uneven proportions, say ¼ potato:¾ lentils, then 75 percent of the glycemic index of the lentils should be added to 25 percent of the glycemic index of potato.

It can be complicated to calculate the precise glycemic index of a combination of foods unless you have access to food composition figures or a nutrient analysis program. As with calories, G.I. values are not as precise a measurement as, for instance, the carat weight of a diamond. Use them simply as a guide.

MAKING THE CHANGE TO A LOW G.I. DIET

Compare thes menus on the following page to see how you could lower the glycemic index of your diet. A simple change can make a big difference.

The Low G.I. Eating Plan has a glycemic index 40 percent **lower** than the High G.I. Eating Plan, plus its fat content is **half** that of the high G.I. menu. Notice how the quantity of food is similar but the calorie content is nearly one-third lower because low fat, high carbohydrate foods have been used.

■ ■ ■

HIGH G.I. EATING PLAN GLYCEMIC INDEX: 67	LOW G.I. EATING PLAN GLYCEMIC INDEX: 41
BREAKFAST	**BREAKFAST**
1 oz. cornflakes and regular milk	1 oz. All Bran with Extra Fiber™ and
2 slices of toast (white bread) with	1% milk
margarine and jam	2 slices toast (whole grain) with
	butter and jam
	An orange
SNACK	**SNACK**
2 sugar cookies	2 oatmeal cookies
LIGHT MEAL	**LIGHT MEAL**
A sandwich (whole wheat bread)	A sandwich (whole grain) with ham
with ham and salad	and salad
A doughnut	Low fat fruit yogurt
SNACK	**SNACK**
Piece of watermelon	An apple
Small bag of potato chips (1 oz.)	Small bag (1 oz.) of peanuts (high fat)
MAIN MEAL	**MAIN MEAL**
Lamb Chops	Small steak
Mashed potato	Pasta with creamy sauce
Carrots	Sweet corn
Peas	Peas
Ice cream	Low fat ice cream
and banana	and peaches
SNACK	**SNACK**
Small bag of corn chips (1 oz.)	Homemade popcorn (3 cups)
ENERGY VALUE:	**ENERGY VALUE:**
2500 Calories	1800 Calories
FAT CONTENT:	**FAT CONTENT:**
120 grams, supplying 44 percent of	60 grams, supplying 28 percent of
energy	energy

BREAKFAST: USING THE GLYCEMIC INDEX TO SUSTAIN YOU THROUGH THE DAY

More and more people these days realize the benefits of having breakfast. Scientifically, having breakfast has been proven to help you lose weight and to lower your cholesterol levels. We also know that eating breakfast can help to stabilize your blood sugar levels. It kick starts your metabolism and gives your body food when it really needs it. Missing breakfast can cause symptoms of fatigue, dehydration and loss of energy. One of the things we notice when non-breakfast eaters start having breakfast is that all of a sudden they develop a morning appetite that they haven't had since childhood. Eating breakfast becomes easier—in fact, it becomes a necessity, which is what it should be. Our bodies require fuel to run on and yet too many of us expect to go about our work without filling up our fuel tank first.

If your breakfast leaves you starving by mid morning, have a closer look at what you ate for breakfast. Many breakfast cereals and breads have a high glycemic index which means while they pick you up initially, they won't last long. When the energy runs out and your blood sugar starts to drop, you feel hungry again. Eating a low G.I. breakfast ensures your breakfast is going to take you through to lunchtime.

In the breakfast section you'll find simple recipes from a quick milkshake to delicious granolas and more adventurous dishes for a weekend breakfast—all guaranteed to sustain you through the day!

A SIMPLE, HEALTHY LOW G.I. BREAKFAST

1. Start with some fruit or juice
Fruit contributes fiber and, more importantly, vitamin C, which helps your body absorb the nutrient iron.

■ ■ ■

LOWEST GLYCEMIC INDEX FRUITS AND JUICES

Cherries	.22	Apple juice (unsweetened)	.40
Grapefruit	.25	Peaches	.42
Dried apricots	.31	Oranges	.44
Apples	.38	Grapes	.46
Pears	.38	Pineapple juice (unsweetened)	.46
Plums	.39	Grapefruit juice (unsweetened)	.48

2. Try some breakfast cereal

Cereals are important as a source of fiber, vitamin B and iron. When choosing processed breakfast cereals, look for those with a high fiber content.

THE TOP SIX IN LOW G.I. CEREALS

Muesli, toasted	.43
Kellogg's Bran Buds with Psyllium™	.45
Old fashioned oats	.49
Kellogg's All Bran with extra fiber™	.51
Kellogg's Special K™	.54
Kellogg's Frosted Flakes™	.55

We know the glycemic index for about twenty brand-name breakfast cereals and, as more research is done, the range of low G.I. cereals will expand.

3. Add milk or yogurt

1% milks and yogurts can make a valuable contribution to your daily calcium intake by including them at breakfast. All have a low glycemic index. Lower fat varieties have just as much, or more, calcium as full cream milk.

4. Plus some bread or toast if you like

■　■　■

LOWEST GLYCEMIC INDEX BREADS

Eagle Mills Bread Mix—soy with flaxseed 50
Pumpernickel (whole grain) 51
Sourdough bread 52
100% stoneground whole wheat . . . . .53 (av)
Eagle Mills Bread Mix—muesli with Sustagrain .54

TEN QUICK LOW FAT, LOW G.I. BREAKFASTS

1. A hot chocolate drink made with low fat milk

2. Toasted 100% stoneground whole wheat bread topped with sliced banana

3. Old fashioned oats sprinkled with raisins and brown sugar

4. A low fat milkshake

5. An 8 ounce container of fat free plain yogurt with sliced peaches and raspberries added

6. Bowl of Bran Buds with Psyllium and 1% milk, topped with unsweetened canned pear slices

7. Low fat American cheese melted on whole grain pumpernickel, topped with a slice of tomato

8. A bowl of All Bran with extra fiber with 1% milk and a glass of freshly squeezed orange juice.

9. Toasted 100% whole wheat pita spread with fresh ricotta or light cream cheese and topped with sliced apple, pear or nectarine.

10. Natural peanut butter on low G.I. toast finished with a piece of fruit.

LUNCH: IDEAS FOR A LIGHT MEAL
OR A G.I. LOWERING SIDE DISH

1. Base your light meals on carbohydrate. Foods such as:

BREAD	PASTA	GRAINS	LEGUMES
bread roll	noodles in soup	steamed rice	baked beans
toast	minestrone	sweet corn	mixed bean salad
sandwiches	fettuccine	tabbouli	curried lentils
fruit loaf	pasta salad	couscous	pea soup
pita bread	ravioli	barley	chili
			chana dal

2. You might add a little meat, cheese, egg, or fish

SIMPLE IDEAS TO ADD		
a sprinkling of Parmesan	hard-boiled egg quarters	sliced boiled ham
sardines and lemon	chopped cooked chicken	sliced turkey breast
a slice of smoked salmon	a cluster of smoked oysters	a sprinkle of bacon bits
a smear of natural peanut butter	8 ozs. of yogurt	a cube of cheddar cheese
a slice of pastrami	tuna (water-packed)	sliced roast beef

Remember—keep the quantity small!

3. Fill it out with vegetables

SIMPLE VEGETABLE IDEAS			
fresh salad greens with vinaigrette	cherry tomatoes	cucumber	grated carrot
	a handful of olives	sliced shallots	shredded cabbage
a spoonful of pesto	crunchy celery sticks	whole baby beets	spinach
a small acorn squash	whole radish	sun-dried tomatoes	pepper strips
snowpeas	cauliflower florets	a sliver of ginger	chopped parsley

4. And round it off with fruit

In the Soups, Salads and Pasta recipe section you'll find ideas for quick, low G.I. lunches plus recipes for substantial salads and soups, (both of which can form a superb start for a low G.I. meal).

LUNCHING OUT

We took a look at some lunch time menus and discovered how to make that takeout lunch a low G.I. choice. Takeout menu items are often high fat, so always consider the fat content of your takeout choices.

LUNCH	OUR ESTIMATED GLYCEMIC INDEX	FAT (GRAMS)
Fresh fruit salad with fat free yogurt	46	Negligible
Fettuccine with tomatoes, olives and garlic (or any other low-fat sauce you care for)	32	8
Go Mexican and choose something with beans, e.g. bean burritos	35	11
Stuffed baked potato with baked beans and cheese	72	12
Thai noodles with vegetables	36	13
Vegetable wrap filled with tabbouli, falafel and salad	48	21
Grilled chicken breast teamed with a small container of bean salad and corn on the cob	39	24
or try Indian... a chicken curry with a little dal and some Basmati rice	48	26

CHANA DAL: THE SUPER-LOW G.I. FOOD

Chana dal, the bean with the lowest glycemic index (G.I.=8), is a diet staple in India, but, as yet, it is still little known in the United States. Scientifically, chana dal is the *desi* type of *Cicer arietinum*. The chana dal bean looks just like yellow split peas, but when cooked, it doesn't readily boil down to mush the way split peas do. It is more closely related to chickpeas (garbanzo beans), but chana dal is younger, smaller, split, sweeter, and has a much lower glycemic index. In fact, you can substitute chana dal for chickpeas in just about any recipe.

Chana dal is generally available in Asian food stores, and as awareness of the value of eating low G.I. foods spreads, it is becoming more widely available. If you don't see it at your favorite food store, ask your local health food store or specialty grocer to carry it.

TEN LOW G.I. LUNCHES ON THE GO

1. Take some pita bread, spread it with hummus, and fill with tabbouli
2. Chunky vegetable soup, thick with barley, beans and macaroni
3. Cook a little pasta and mix through pesto, or chopped fresh herbs or sundried tomatoes
4. Put your favorite sandwich filling on whole grain bread (a grilled sandwich if you like)
5. Beat up a banana smoothie and couple it with a high fiber apple muffin
6. Mix fresh fruit with nonfat yogurt
7. Take a green salad with vinaigrette dressing plus some bean salad, add whole grain bread and enjoy!
8. Stir-fry tofu, Chinese vegetables and noodles
9. Smoked salmon on pumpernickel with avocado
10. Veggie burger with grilled vegetables on a whole wheat sandwich bun

MAIN MEALS: CHOOSING THE BEST WITH LOW G.I.

What to make for dinner is the perennial question. When organizing the ingredients in your mind for a main meal, think of them appearing in the following order.

1. First choose the carbohydrate

Which will it be? Potato, rice, pasta, grains, legumes or a combination? Could you add some bread or corn? See below for further help.

CHOOSING YOUR MAIN MEAL CARBOHYDRATE

It isn't just a matter of choosing the food with the lowest glycemic index. It is best to include a wide variety of foods in your diet to optimize your nutrient intake. Compare the nutritional properties of these carbohydrate foods and see why variety is important.

New potatoes Potatoes are a good source of vitamin C and potassium. The content of both these nutrients is higher when less water and shorter cooking times are used in the preparation of potatoes. Potatoes themselves do not contain fat so think twice about how you cook them. Just remember that new potatoes have the lowest glycemic index at 56, and other varieties have a higher glycemic index.

Rice White rice is bland in flavor, making it an ideal accompaniment to spicy Chinese, Thai, Vietnamese, and Indian food. Milling of rice removes the bran and germ, resulting in a considerable loss of nutrients. Because of this, brown rice is a much better source of B vitamins, minerals and fiber. Vary your diet to include both brown and white rice.

Sweet potato Orange sweet potato is a fantastic source of beta-carotene (the plant precursor of vitamin A) and is also quite rich in vitamin C and makes a colorful addition to any dinner. It is a good source of fiber. Its glycemic index is 54.

Sweet corn Corn on the cob, or loose kernel corn, or cream style corn is generally a popular vegetable with children and is high in fiber. It is also a source of B vitamins. Its glycemic index is 55.

Legumes Chickpeas, lentils and beans are all high in protein and so are a nutritious alternative to meat. Their content of niacin, potassium, phosphorus, iron and zinc is also high, while their fiber content is higher than for the other carbohydrate foods listed here. Their glycemic index varies—check the tables at back of book.

Pasta Pasta is higher in protein than rice or potato and is often eaten as a meal without including meat. It is very satisfying and quick to prepare with the addition of vegetables, or a

	vegetable sauce and a sprinkling of Parmesan. Its glycemic index varies from 37 to 55.
Cracked wheat	Bulgur (burghul) is parboiled whole or cracked grains of wheat. Because the whole grain is virtually intact, bulgur provides lots of fiber, thiamin, niacin, vitamin E and minerals. Its glycemic index is 48.

2. Add vegetables—and lots of them

Fresh, frozen, canned—whatever you have, the more the merrier. Refer to the vegetables list under lunches for inspiration, or use your favorites. Think of a bowl of crisp salad with a sprinkling of chopped sun-dried tomatoes plus 1 tablespoon Vinaigrette dressing.

3. Just a little protein for flavor and texture

Remember, we don't need much—some slivers of beef to stir-fry, a sprinkle of tasty cheese, strips of ham, a dollop of ricotta, a tender chicken breast, slices of salmon, a couple of eggs, a handful of nuts, or use the protein found in your grains and legumes.

4. Think twice about using any fat

Check that you are using a healthy type (a monounsaturated or a polyunsaturated) and reduce the quantity if you can.

The following pages are packed with ideas on how to create a low fat, G.I. meal in minutes.

TEN LOW G.I. MAIN MEALS IN MINUTES

1. Speedy Spaghetti

Bring a large pot of water to the boil, add the spaghetti and cook according to the directions on the packet. Meanwhile, open a jar of chunky tomato sauce and heat. Make a green salad with lettuce, spring onions and cucumber or a bag of mixed lettuce. Serve the spaghetti, topped with the pasta sauce, a good sprinkle of Parmesan cheese and a green salad with vinaigrette alongside.

■ ■ ■

2. Fast Fish and Tiny 'Taters

Take a boneless fillet of fresh fish. Dust it with seasoned flour. Heat a non-stick pan with a film of oil and pop the fish in to fry. Wash a handful of tiny new potatoes and microwave or steam them until tender. Squeeze lemon juice over the fish once you have cooked both sides and sprinkle with pepper. Serve immediately with the potatoes and a salad or mixed vegetables.

3. Quick Pita Pizza

Spread a 2 ounce round of pita bread with pesto or tomato paste. Top with sliced tomato, mushrooms, roasted peppers, black olives, chopped spring onions or scallions and a sprinkle of Parmesan cheese. Heat through under the broiler or in a hot oven.

4. Oriental Noodle and Vegetable Stir-Fry

Stir-fry 2 strips of diced bacon (all fat removed) or ham. Add a package of oriental stir-fry frozen vegetable mix, cooking according to the directions on the bag. Mix in some fresh egg noodles or prepared instant noodles a few minutes before the end of cooking time and heat through before serving.

   Tip Look for the bags of frozen stir-fry vegetable mixes that have
   noodles and a sauce packet included.

5. Time-saving Tortellini

Boil a package of spinach and cheese (or your favorite filling) tortellini according to package directions. Heat some bottled tomato pasta sauce and serve this on top of the tortellini with a sprinkle of Parmesan cheese. Add a salad and vinaigrette alongside.

6. Racey Rice and Lentils

Boil some Basmati or Uncle Ben's Converted rice. Heat a heavy-based frypan with a little oil. Add a finely diced onion, crushed garlic and a couple of teaspoons of minced chili. Saute until the onion is soft. Meanwhile dice a tomato and mix with the onion. Open a can of lentil soup and add to the pan. Add ground cumin, salt and pepper to season, heat through and serve alongside the rice.

7. Easy Chicken Pasta

Boil 4 ounces of shell pasta. Meanwhile, thinly slice half a red pepper, a handful of button mushrooms and a stalk of celery. Chop some leftover barbeque chicken into bite-size pieces. Drain the pasta, add the pepper, mushrooms, celery and chicken and pour over some light creamy salad dressing. Top with chopped spring onions or scallions and serve.

8. Tomato and Tuna Pasta

Boil some pasta. In a small pan saute some chopped parsley, garlic and chili (optional) in a little oil until aromatic. Add a can of chopped tomatoes (undrained) and small can of flaked tuna. Season with pepper and heat through. Serve the tuna and tomato sauce over pasta.

9. Mexican in Minutes

Brown a handful of lean ground beef and a finely diced onion in a pan. Add a small can of Heinz Mexi Beans and taco seasoning if desired. Heat through. Serve with tomato salsa, shredded lettuce, avocado and grated cheese in taco shells or pita bread.

10. Quick Thai Noodle Curry

Stir-fry some strips of onion, red pepper, baby corn and snow peas (or any stir-fry vegetable mix) in a large pan or wok. Add a tablespoon of red curry paste. Prepare a packet of instant noodles according to directions. Add the noodles to the vegetables with enough of the liquid to make a sauce. Stir in a tablespoon of coconut milk, heat through and it's ready to serve.

Tip Canned coconut milk or cream, can be poured into ice-block trays, frozen and then kept in a plastic bag, making it easy to add just a tablespoon to a dish. Alternatively coconut milk powder can be kept in the pantry and mixed as needed.

■ ■ ■

DESSERTS: A LOW G.I. FINISH

It's fairly easy to give a meal a low G.I. twist through dessert. This is because many of the basic components of dessert, like fruit and dairy products, have a low glycemic index.

In discussions with people about what they eat these days, dessert is seldom mentioned. With busier lifestyles and concerns about being overweight, dessert is conveniently missed. While this appears a positive change in eliminating unnecessary calories from the diet, there is a negative side. In many instances desserts can make a valuable contribution to our daily calcium and vitamin C intakes because they are frequently based on dairy foods and fruits. What's more, desserts are usually carbohydrate rich, which means they help top-up our satiety levels and thereby signify the completion of eating.

The basis of a perfect dessert—low G.I. fruits and dairy foods

Citrus   A winter fruit which is an excellent source of vitamin C. Select heavy fruit with fine textured glossy skin. Oranges are good as a snack cut into quarters and frozen. Soak segments of a variety of citrus fruit in orange juice with a slurp of brandy, scatter with raisins and serve as winter fruit salad.

Cherries   A true summer fruit. Choose plump fruit, bright red/black color on fresh green stems. A bowl of cherries on the table is a lovely dessert to share.

Stone fruits   Apricots appear earliest in the season. Choose those with as much golden orange color as possible, avoiding pale or green fruit. Peaches and nectarines should be just beginning to soften. Fresh sliced peaches or nectarines are delicious with ice cream or yogurt. Sprinkle fresh peach halves with cinnamon and try them lightly broiled or stewed.

Pears and apples   At their peak during autumn and winter, but are available all year. Preparation simply involves washing and slicing and they provide the perfect finish to a meal.

Grapes One of the most popular fruits with children because they are so sweet and easy to eat. Grapes do not ripen after harvest so choose bunches with a deep, uniform color on fresh green stems. Put a bowl on the table after a meal or include them in a fruit salad.

Pudding, ice cream and yogurt Look for low fat or fat free varieties for a cool and creamy treat.

SOMETHING SWEET

Sugar or sucrose, a common ingredient in traditional desserts, has a glycemic index of 65. Most sugary foods have low-to-moderate G.I. values. Cakes and cookies made with or without sugar have similar G.I. values. Recipes incorporating fruit for sweetness rather than sugar, will have more fiber and a lower G.I. Remember temperate-climate fruits such as apples, pears and stone fruits tend to have the lowest glycemic index values.

EIGHT QUICK AND EASY LOW G.I. DESSERTS

1. Low fat ice cream and strawberries

2. Baked whole apple, stuffed with dried fruit

3. Fruit salad with low fat yogurt

4. Make a fruit crumble—top cooked fruit with a crumbled mixture of toasted muesli, wheat flakes, a little melted butter, and honey

5. Slice a firm banana into some low fat pudding

6. Top unsweetened canned fruit (peaches or pears) with low fat ice cream or low fat pudding or sugar free Jello-O

7. Wrap chopped apple, raisins, currants and spice in a sheet of filo pastry (brushed with milk, not fat) and bake as a strudel

8. Low fat fruit yogurt

SNACKS: KEEPING YOUR ENERGY LEVELS UP BETWEEN MEALS

The fine art of grazing! Hands up all those who thought that sensible eating meant keeping to three meals a day? Traditionally, there has been a belief that sensible eating meant sticking to three square meals a day. Perhaps this stems from images of an erratic eater. You know the one, the person who skips breakfast making up for it with snacks during the day and then feasting before sleeping at night—certainly not the ideal pattern! New evidence suggests that the people who graze properly, eating small amounts of food throughout the day at frequent intervals, may actually be doing themselves a favor.

A recent study which compared people eating a diet of three meals a day with those who had three meals and three snacks showed that snacking stimulated the body to use up more energy for metabolism compared to concentrating the same amount of food into three meals. It's as if the more fuel you give your body the more it will burn. Frequent small meals stimulate the metabolic rate.

The problem with grazing is that most snacks turn out to be high fat foods like cakes, chocolate, snack bars, chips or pastries. Another criticism of grazing has been that for people who eat too much, increasing the number of times that they face food is tempting disaster. Overeating is less likely to occur if the foods eaten are carbohydrate rich and have a low glycemic index. Using these foods, you will feel satisfied before you have overconsumed!

SUSTAINING SNACKS

Try a muffin
A smoothie
100% stoneground whole wheat raisin toast

A juicy orange
A small can of baked beans
A bowl of All Bran™ with 1% milk
A piece of pita bread with hummus
A small container of low fat yogurt
A sandwich
Dried apricots
A handful of raisins
A big green apple
Low fat ice cream in a cone
3 cups of popcorn (low fat of course)

Chapter 11

COOKING THE LOW G.I. WAY

HOW YOU CAN REDUCE THE GLYCEMIC INDEX OF
RECIPES AND MEALS

THE A TO Z REDUCING THE FAT CONTENT
OF A RECIPE

THE LOW G.I. PANTRY

WHAT TO KEEP IN THE REFRIGERATOR AND FREEZER

THE LOW G.I. FOOD GLOSSARY

Many of your favorite recipes can be modified to lower their glycemic index value. The first step is to become familiar with the glycemic index of a range of foods. Take a critical look at your meals and consider how you could reduce the glycemic index. Perhaps you could try All Bran or Bran Buds with Psyllium for breakfast instead of cornflakes or Rice Krispies? At lunch time you could ask for a sandwich made from a bread based on whole grains instead of refined flour. For your evening meal, why not have pasta instead of potato and add some other low G.I. ingredients like legumes, sweet corn or peas?

Changing one ingredient in a recipe can be enough to lower the glycemic index of the final dish. The more low G.I. food(s) in the recipe the greater the effect and the lower the overall glycemic index. If the recipe is based on high G.I. ingredients and you feel it can't be changed, try serving it with some low G.I. accompaniments.

HOW YOU CAN REDUCE THE GLYCEMIC INDEX
OF RECIPES AND MEALS

IN PLACE OF:	LOW G.I. ALTERNATIVE
Bread	Substitute about 50% of the flour with whole or cracked grains. Alvarado Farms, Shiloh Farms, Wild and Vermont Bread Company are good commercial brands.
Flour	In baked goods, reduce the amount of flour, partially substituting with oat bran, rice bran, or rolled oats
Rice	Try Basmati or Uncle Ben's Converted™ rice, or pearled barley, quick-cooking wheat, buckwheat, bulgur, couscous or instant noodles
Potato	Sweet potato, new potatoes, Basmati rice, pasta, sweet corn
Sugar	Try apple juice or dried fruit to sweeten. Honey also has a slightly lower G.I.
Bananas, mango, papaya, oranges, pineapple, canteloupe, and other tropical fruits have higher G.I. levels	Try apples, cherries, grapefruit, peaches, pears, plums, and other temperate-climate fruits more often— or combine them with a higher G.I. fruit

■ ■ ■

IN RECIPES FOR	LOW G.I. ALTERNATIVE
Soups	Add lentils, barley, split peas, navy beans and pasta—make a minestrone!
Casseroles	Try substituting kidney beans, pinto beans or lentils for a portion of the meat. Boosts the fiber and drops the fat too!
Meatballs or meat loaf	Add cooked lentils, canned beans, or rolled oats in combination with the ground beef.

HOW TO LOWER THE G.I. OF A RECIPE WHILE KEEPING THE NUTRITION HIGH

Take a recipe such as:

Plain Cup Cakes

1 egg

1 cup milk

½ cup sugar

2 cups flour

1 tablespoon baking powder

4 ozs. (1 stick) butter

The bulk of this recipe is flour (a high G.I. ingredient) plus sugar (an ingredient of intermediate G.I. value). The glycemic index of the recipe is 67.

- The first step is to reduce the amount of flour, partially substituting with a lower G.I. food, like oat bran.
- The next step is to see if some of the intermediate G.I. ingredients can be substituted for ingredients with a lower G.I. Sugar can be partially replaced with fruit or fruit juice, for example.
- The resulting recipe—a combination of high G.I. ingredients with low G.I. ingredients—gives us a product with a lower total G.I. value.

So, putting some changes into place:

(adding low G.I. fruit for flavor and fiber)	1 coarsely grated apple
	1 egg
	½ cup 1% or skim milk
(using foods with a lower G.I. for sweetness)	½ cup apple juice
	⅓ cup raisins
(reducing the amount of flour)	1 cup flour
	½ tablespoon baking powder
(substituting oat bran for flour)	½ cup unprocessed oat bran
(reduced amount of butter)	2 ozs. (½ stick) butter

The finished product: Apple Raisin Muffins which are lower in fat, higher in fiber and have a glycemic index 10 points lower than the original recipe at 59.

THE A TO Z OF REDUCING THE FAT
CONTENT OF A RECIPE

As we have said constantly throughout this book, it is important to eat a high carbohydrate and low fat diet. The following practical tips which we have set out in an easy A to Z format will help you reduce the fat content of some of your favorite recipes at the same time as you are lowering their glycemic index.

Alcohol Although excessive alcohol consumption can be fattening, as an ingredient in a recipe, alcohol itself won't create a high calorie dish. Alcohol evaporates during cooking, so you lose the calories and are left with the flavor. A little wine in a sauce can give a delicious flavor, and sherry in an Asian style marinade is essential.

Bacon Bacon is a valuable ingredient in many dishes because of the flavor it offers. You can make a little bacon go a long way by trimming off all fat and chopping it finely. Lean ham is often a more economical and leaner way to go. In casseroles and soups, a ham or bacon bone imparts a fine flavor without much fat.

Cheese At around 30 percent fat (23 percent of this being saturated), cheese can contribute quite a lot of fat to a recipe. Although there are a number of fat-reduced cheeses available, many of these lose a lot in flavor for a small reduction in fat. It is worth comparing fat per ounce between brands to find the tastiest one with the lowest fat content. Alternatively, a sprinkle of a grated, very tasty cheese or Parmesan, may do the job.

Part skim ricotta and cottage cheeses are lower fat alternatives to butter on a sandwich. It's worth trying some fresh part skim ricotta from a deli—you may find the texture and flavor more acceptable than that of the ricotta available in containers in the supermarket. Flavored cottage cheeses are ideal low fat toppings for crackers. Try ricotta in lasagna instead of a creamy white sauce.

Cream and sour cream Keep to very small amounts as these are high in saturated fat. Substitute nonfat sour cream, which tastes very similar to the full fat variety. A 16 ounce container of heavy cream can be poured into ice-cube trays and frozen providing small servings of cream easily when you need it. Adding one ice-cube block (1 ounce) of cream to a dish adds only 5.5 grams of fat.

Dried beans, peas and lentils These are all low in fat and very nutritious. Incorporating them in a recipe, perhaps as partial substitution of meat, will lower the fat content of the finished product. Canned beans, chick peas and lentils are now widely available. They are very convenient to use and a great time saver. They are comparable in food value to the dried ones that you soak and cook yourself.

Eggs Be conscious of eggs in a recipe as they can add fat. Sometimes just the beaten egg white can be substituted for the whole egg, or use real egg substitute.

Filo pastry Unlike most other pastry, filo is low in fat. To keep it that way brush between the sheets with skim milk instead of melted butter when you prepare it. Look for it in the freezer section of the supermarket with other prepared pastry and use it as a pie topping or a strudel wrap.

Grilling Grill or broil tender cuts of meat, chicken and fish rather than fry. Marinating first will add flavor, moisture and tenderness.

Health food stores Health food stores can be traps for the unwary. Check out the high fat ingredients, such as hydrogenated vegetable oil, nuts, coconut and palm kernel oil in the products such as granola bars, fruit bars, and "health" cakes (even if made with whole wheat flour) that they stock on their shelves.

Ice cream A source of carbohydrate, calcium, riboflavin, retinol and protein and low fat varieties have the lower glycemic index—definitely a nutritious and icy treat.

Jam A tablespoon of jam on toast contains far fewer calories than a pat of butter on toast. So, enjoy your jam and give fat the flick!

Keep jars of minced garlic, chili or ginger in the refrigerator to spice up your cooking in an instant.

Lemon juice Try a fresh squeeze with ground black pepper on vegetables rather than a pat of butter. Lemon juice provides acidity that slows gastric emptying and lowers the G.I.

Milk Many people dislike skim milk, particularly when they taste it on its own or in their coffee! However, you can use skim milk in a recipe and no one will notice—and the fat saving is great. For convenience you might want to keep powdered skim milk in the pantry, which can be made up to the desired quantity when you need it. It will taste more like fresh milk if you mix the powder and water according to directions and refrigerate the milk overnight before using it. Ultra-pasteurized milk is handy in the cupboard, too.

Nuts They are valuable for their content of vitamin E, but they are also high in fat. To keep the fat content of a recipe low, the quantity of nuts has to be small.

Oil Most of our recipes call for no more than 2 teaspoons of oil. Any polyunsaturated or monounsaturated oil is suitable. Cooking spray or brushing oil lightly over the base of the pan is ideal. If you find the amount of oil insufficient, cover your pan, or add a few drops of water and use steam to cook the ingredients without burning. It is a good idea to invest in a nonstick frying pan if you don't have one!

Pasta A food to eat more of and a great source of carbohydrate and B vitamins. Fresh or dried, the preparation is easy. Just boil in water until just tender or "al dente," drain and top with a dollop of pesto, a tomato sauce or a sprinkle of Parmesan and pepper. There are many wonderful pasta cookbooks now available. It is definitely worth investing in one to find all sorts of exciting ways to prepare this fabulous low G.I. food. Pasta may appear in your menu as a side dish to meat, as noodles in soup, as a meal in itself with vegetables or sauce or even as an ingredient in a dessert.

Questions Ask your dietitian for more recipe ideas. (See page 15 for guidance on finding one.)

Reduce the fat content of ground beef by browning it in a nonstick pan, then placing the meat in a colander and pouring boiling water through it to wash away the fat. Return to the pan to continue cooking. It is a good idea to buy the better quality ground beef with less fat.

Stock If you are prepared to go to the effort of making your own stock—good for you! Prepare it in advance, refrigerate it then skim off the accumulated fat from the top. Prepared stock is available in long-life cartons in the supermarket. Stock cubes are another alternative. Look for brands that have reduced salt.

To sauté Heat the pan first, brush with the recommended amount of oil or less, add the food and cook, stirring lightly over a gentle heat.

Underlying the need for fat is a need for taste. Be creative with other flavorings.

Vinegar A vinaigrette dressing (1 tablespoon vinegar and 2 teaspoons of oil) with your salad can lower the blood sugar response to the whole meal by up to 30 percent. The best types of vinegars for this purpose are red or white wine vinegar, or use lemon juice.

Weighing What's the weight of the meat you're buying? Start noticing the weight that appears on the butcher's scales or package label and consider how many servings it will give you. With something like steak, that is basically all edible meat, 4–5 ounces per serving is sufficient. One pound is more than enough for four portions. Choose lean cuts of meat. Trim the fat off before cooking or before you put it away. Alternate meat or chicken with fish once or twice a week.

Yogurt Yogurt is a valuable food in many ways. It is a good source of calcium, and "friendly bacteria," protein and riboflavin and unlike milk, is suitable for those who are lactose intolerant. Low fat plain yogurt is a suitable substitute for sour cream. If using yogurt in a hot sauce or casserole, add it at the last minute and do not let it boil, or it will curdle. It is best if you can bring the yogurt to room temperature before adding to the hot dish. To do this, mix a small amount of yogurt with a little sauce from the dish, then stir this mixture back into the bulk of the sauce.

Zero fat Eating zero fat is unhealthy, so speak with a dietitian about how to get just the right amount you need. Our bodies need essential fatty acids that can't be sythesized and must be supplied in the diet. Fat does add flavor—use it to your advantage.

■ ■ ■

THE LOW G.I. PANTRY

To make low G.I. choices *easy* choices, you need to keep the right foods in your pantry.

None of the following breads are made with refined enriched flour; rather, they are made from whole grain flours.
   Alvarado Farms 100% Sprouted Wheat
   Arnold Stoneground 100% Whole Wheat
   Braunschlagger European Style Rye
   Martins Dutch Country 100% Stoneground Whole Wheat
      Sandwich Roll
   Pepperidge Farm Sprouted Wheat™
   Pritikin Whole Grain Whole Wheat Rye™
   Shiloh Farms Cracked Wheat, 100% Whole Grain Wheat
   Shra Lins Greek Style Whole Wheat Pita
   Taystee 100% Stoneground Whole Wheat
   Toufayan's 100% Whole Wheat Pita
   Vermont Bread Company 100% Whole Wheat, Alfalfa Sprouts,
      Sprouted Wheat, etc.
   Wild's Whole Grain
   Wonder Stoneground 100% Whole Wheat
Cereals
   Kellogg's All-Bran with extra fiber™
   Kellogg's Bran Buds with Psyllium™
   Muesli (low fat varieties, read the labels)
   Rolled oats
   Oat bran
   Rice bran
   Pearled barley
   Basmati rice
   Uncle Ben's Converted™ Rice
   Pasta of various shapes and flavors
Canned or dried lentils (red and brown), legumes (chickpeas,
   cannellini beans)
A variety of canned legumes (kidney beans, chickpeas, cannellini
   beans, black beans, pinto beans, butter beans, broad beans,
   baked beans)

Canned sweet corn. Other canned vegetables like canned tomatoes, asparagus, peas, mushrooms are always handy to boost the vegetable content of a meal

Tomato paste

Canned crushed tomatoes and tomato puree, bottled tomato pasta sauces

Prepared chicken stock, e.g. Campbell's "Real Stock" or bouillon cubes

Low oil salad dressings and vinaigrette

Dried fruits—raisins, dried apricots, fruit medley, raisins, prunes etc.

Canned peaches, pears, apple

Long-life skim milk or skim milk powder

Canned evaporated skim milk

Pudding mixes, cooked not instant

Spices—curry powder, cumin, turmeric, mustard etc.

Herbs—oregano, basil, thyme are the most used in these recipes. Pre-mixed blends of these are available

Bottled minced ginger, chili and garlic

WHAT TO KEEP IN THE REFRIGERATOR AND FREEZER

Skim or 1% milk
Low fat plain yogurt
Low fat fruit yogurt
Low fat ice cream
Frozen low fat yogurt, sorbet, gelato
Eggs
Cheese
   low fat processed slices
   reduced fat or low fat cheddar
   grated Parmesan
   1% cottage or part skim ricotta cheese
Frozen peas and corn
Frozen berries

■ ■ ■

THE LOW G.I. FOOD GLOSSARY

This glossary describes some of the key foods that can form part of a low G.I. diet.

Apples (G.I. of 38) • Easy-to-incorporate into the diet as a low G.I. food—an average apple will add 3 grams of fiber to your diet. They are also high in pectin, which lowers their glycemic index.

Apple juice (G.I. of 40) • The main sugar occurring in apples is fructose (6.5 percent) which itself has a low G.I. The high concentration of sugars is known to slow the rate of stomach emptying, hence slowing the absorption and lowering G.I.

Apricots (G.I. of 64, canned; 31, dried) • Apricots are an excellent source of beta-carotene and dried apricots in particular are high in potassium. Like apples, they are high in fructose (5.1 percent) which lowers their G.I.

Barley (G.I. of 25) • "Pearled" barley, which has had the outer brown layers removed, is most commonly used. It is high in soluble fiber which probably contributes to its low G.I. Available in supermarkets.

Basmati rice (G.I. of 58) • Has a low G.I. attributable to the type of starch it contains (high amylose starch). Available in supermarkets.

Breakfast cereals • The high degree of cooking and processing of commercial breakfast cereals tends to make the starch in them more rapidly digestible, giving a higher G.I. Less processed cereals (muesli, rolled oats) tend to have lower G.I. values. Kellogg's All-Bran (G.I. of 42) although processed, is not made from milled starch but large flakes of raw bran.

Buckwheat (G.I. of 54) • Buckwheat is available from health food stores and some supermarkets. It can be cooked like oatmeal or steamed and served with vegetables, in place of rice. It can also be ground and used as flour for making pancakes and pasta. Buckwheat in this form is likely to have a higher G.I. than when whole.

Bulgur (G.I. of 48) • Is made by roughly grinding previously cooked and dried wheat. Most commonly recognized as a main ingredient in tabouli. The intact physical form of the wheat contributes to its low G.I.

Cherries (G.I. of 22) • The glycemic index for cherries is based on a study of German cherries, which are often very sour. American cherries are less acidic and their glycemic index may be correspondingly higher, although still within the low G.I. range.

Grapefruit (G.I. of 25) • The low glycemic index of grapefruit may be due to their high acid content which slows absorption from the stomach.

Grapes (G.I. of 46) • An equal mix of fructose and glucose and a high acid content are characteristics of fruits with a low G.I. Grapes are a good example.

Ice cream (G.I. of 61) • Most dairy products have very low glycemic index values. When we eat dairy foods a protein curd forms in the stomach and slows down its emptying. This has the effect of slowing down absorption and lowering the glycemic index.

Kiwi (G.I. of 52) • Kiwi contain equal proportions of glucose and fructose and high acidity giving a reasonably low G.I. They are also a wonderful source of vitamin C with one kiwi meeting the total recommended daily intake.

Legumes (G.I. range: 14 to 56) • These include dried peas, beans and lentils, and mostly have a glycemic index of 50 or less. Canned varieties have a slightly higher G.I. than their home-cooked counterpart due to the higher temperature during processing. Soy beans (G.I. of 18) have one of the lowest G.I. values, possibly due to their higher protein and fat content. The viscous fiber in legumes reduces physical availability of starch to digestive enzymes.

Lemon juice (G.I. = 0) • A small amount of lemon juice (1 tablespoon) won't add any carbohydrate but its acidity has a powerful slowing effect on stomach emptying, thereby slowing down the rate of starch digestion. Vinegar has the same effect.

Milk (G.I. of 27) • Lactose, the sugar occurring naturally in milk, is a disaccharide which must be digested into its component sugars before absorption. The two sugars that result, glucose and galactose, compete with each other for absorption. This slows down absorption and lowers the G.I. The presence of protein and fat in milk also lowers the G.I. of milk.

Oat bran (G.I. of 55) • Unprocessed oat bran is available in the cereal section of supermarkets, usually loosely packed in plastic bags. Its carbohydrate content is lower than that of oats and it is higher in fiber, particularly soluble fiber, which is probably responsible for its low G.I. A soft, bland product, it is useful as a partial substitution for flour in baked goods to lower the G.I.

Oatmeal • Published glycemic index values range from a low 42 up to 66 for "one minute oats." The additional cutting of rolled oats to produce quick cooking oats probably increases the rate of digestion causing a higher G.I.

Oranges (G.I. of 44) • Well known as a good source of vitamin C, most of the sugar content of oranges is sucrose. This, and their high acid content, probably accounts for their low G.I.

Parboiled (minute) rice (G.I. range: 38 to 87) • Parboiling involves steeping rice in hot water and steaming it prior to drying and milling. Nutrients from the bran layer are retained in the grain and the cooked product has less tendency to be sticky. The overriding determinant of the G.I. of rice is the type of starch present in the grain.

Pasta (G.I. range: 32 to 64) • Pasta is made from hard wheat semolina with a high protein content, which gives a strong dough. Protein-starch interactions and minimal disruption to the starch granules during processing contribute to the low G.I. There is some evidence that thicker pasta has a lower G.I. than thin types.

Peach (G.I. of 42, fresh; 30, canned) • Most of the sugar in peaches is sucrose (4.7 percent). Other aspects like their acid and fiber content may account for their low G.I.

Peanuts (G.I. of 14) • A low carbohydrate but high fat food, being 50 percent fat and 25 percent protein, which is one reason for the low G.I. value.

Pear (G.I. of 38, fresh; 44, canned) • Another fruit with a high fructose (6.7 percent) content, accounting for the low G.I.

Peas (G.I. of 48) • Peas are high in fiber and also higher in protein than most other vegetables. Protein-starch interactions may contribute to their lower G.I. They also average 3.5 percent sucrose giving them a sweet flavor.

Pineapple juice (G.I. of 46) • Mainly sucrose (7.9 percent).

Pita bread (G.I. of 57) • Unleavened flat bread was found to have a slightly lower G.I. than regular bread in a Canadian study. Sold in supermarkets in package of flat rounds.

Plums (G.I. of 39) • The G.I. for plums comes from a European study. Australian plums contain a fairly equal mixture of glucose, fructose and sucrose. The higher the concentration of sugars, the slower the food is emptied from the stomach and hence the slower the absorption. This may account for the low G.I.

Popcorn (G.I. of 55) • A surprisingly low G.I. for a processed product. The type of starch or changes to its structure in the popping and cooling of the popcorn may be the cause of the lower G.I. Popcorn is a high fiber snack food.

Potatoes, new (G.I. of 56) • These potatoes are small with white skin. They have a lower glycemic index than other potatoes and the reason why is their starch is more difficult to gelatinize.

Pudding (G.I. of 43) • Pudding is made with milk, so it provides calcium, protein and B vitamins plus a little sugar, vanilla flavoring and a starch thickener.

Pumpernickel bread (G.I. of 41) • Also known as rye kernel bread because the dough it is made from contains 80 to 90 percent whole rye kernels. It has a strong flavor and is usually sold thinly sliced. Because it is not made with fine flour, its G.I. is much lower than ordinary bread. Available in supermarkets and delicatessens.

Rice bran (G.I. of 19) • Rich in fiber (25 percent by weight) and oil (20 percent by weight), rice bran has an extremely low G.I. It is available in the cereal section of supermarkets.

Spaghetti (G.I. of 41) • While both fresh and dried pastas have a low G.I., this is not the case for canned spaghetti. Canned spaghetti is generally made from flour rather than high protein semolina and is very well cooked—two factors which are likely to give it a high G.I.

Sweet corn (G.I. of 55) • Raw, fresh, frozen or canned varieties would be suitable to use. Corn on the cob has a lower G.I. than corn chips or cornflakes. The intact whole kernel makes enzymic attack more difficult.

Sweet potato (G.I. of 54) • Belonging to a different plant family from regular potato, sweet potatoes are mainly available either white or yellow/orange in color. The "sweetness" comes from a high sucrose content. Sweet potato is high in fiber. It has a lower G.I. than regular potato varieties.

Vinegar (G.I. = 0) • All types of vinegars, even in small amounts (1 tablespoon) contain acids which put a break on stomach emptying and slow down digestion in the small intestine. The most effective appear to be red and white wine vinegars.

Yogurt (G.I. of 33) • A concentrated milk product, soured by the use of specific bacteria. All varieties have a low G.I, including those that contain fruit and/or sugar. Artificially sweetened brands have both a lower glycemic index and contain fewer calories than naturally sweetened yogurt.

Chapter 12

THE RECIPES

BREAKFASTS

SOUPS

SALADS

PASTAS

MAIN DISHES

SIDE DISHES

DESSERTS

SNACKS

*L*ow G.I. eating means making a move back to the high carbohydrate foods which are staples in many parts of the
world. The emphasis is on whole foods like whole grains—
barley, oats, dried peas and beans, in combination with certain types
of rice, breads, pasta, vegetables and fruits. You'll find the recipes
listed under each of our three main eating occasions—breakfasts,
light meals (like soups, salads and pastas), and main meals, with
additional sections on desserts and snacks. While some of the recipes
are specifically modified to lower the G.I., others are included to present new ways of preparing low G.I. foods.

The recipes have been developed to help you reduce the overall
glycemic index of your diet, improving its nutritional quality while
you do it. They are designed to be incorporated into your usual diet,
helping you to get your carbohydrate intake up to 50 to 60 percent
of your calorie intake and keeping your fat intake down to the recommended level of 30 percent of calories per day. Protein should

stay constant at 10 to 15 percent of energy. Most of the recipes are high in fiber, both soluble and insoluble. Salt has been added where necessary for flavor, but may be omitted according to taste.

Each recipe has been analyzed for its nutritional value which is given per serving where the recipe is divided into a specified number of servings. The following information will help put this nutritional profile into context for you.

Calories. This is the measure of how much energy the food provides. Those who burn lots of energy through exercise need a higher calorie intake than those who live more sedentary lives. A moderately active woman aged 18 to 54 years would consume about 1800 calories a day; a man about 2300 calories.

Fat Our fat requirement is probably as small as 10 grams (equivalent to 2 ½ teaspoons butter) a day to provide essential fatty acids needed for health. The range of acceptable fat intake depends on your total calorie intake. People trying to lose weight could aim for around 30 to 40 grams (7–10 teaspoons of butter) of fat a day. Most others could do with 50 to 60 grams (12–15 teaspoons of butter). Children and adolescents need more than adults because they are growing and should not have their fat intake overly restricted.

Carbohydrate The total amount of carbohydrate (which includes starches and sugars) is listed with each recipe. Our aim is to help you increase your carbohydrate intake as your fat intake drops. It is not necessary to calculate how many grams of carbohydrate you eat on a daily basis, however the athlete or person with diabetes may find this information useful. This is so they can eat enough! On average, women should take in 250 grams of carbohydrate (equivalent to 16 slices of bread) each day while men need about 350 grams (23 slices of bread). Athletes can consume anywhere from 350 to 700 grams of carbohydrate a day (23–47 slices of bread).

Fiber It is recommended that we consume at least 30 grams of dietary fiber every day. A slice of whole grain bread provides 2 grams of fiber, an average apple 4 grams. The average American consumes only 11 grams of fiber a day.

Breakfasts

BREAKFAST IN A GLASS

GOLDEN PLUM GRANOLA

CREAMY OATMEAL WITH BANANA AND RAISINS

FRUIT 'N' OAT HOTCAKES

BUTTERMILK PANCAKES WITH FRUIT

MUSHROOM CHEESE OMELET

CRISPY TOAST AND TOMATOES

■

Breakfast in a Glass

The "smoothie"—a quick, but sustaining breakfast. Many variations are possible using different combinations of fruits, milks and yogurts.

■

GLYCEMIC INDEX: 49
NUTRIENTS PER SERVING:

CALORIES 191
FAT . . . . .2 g
CARBOHYDRATE . . . . .35 g
FIBER . . . . .2 g

1. Peel banana and chop coarsely

2. Combine with remaining ingredients in a blender and blend for 30 seconds or until smooth and thick.

3. Serve immediately.

SERVES 2

Note: The 4 ozs. of evaporated nonfat milk and the 8 ozs. 1% milk can be substituted with 4 ozs. 1% milk and 8 ozs. nonfat plain yogurt.

1 large, ripe banana (about 5 ozs.)

1 cup (8 ozs.) 1% milk, chilled

½ cup (4 ozs.) evaporated nonfat milk, well chilled

2 teaspoons honey

few drops vanilla extract

For this recipe the evaporated milk must be chilled to froth up well.

Golden Plum Granola

Because this breakfast is nutritionally power-packed, a little goes a long way. In a closed container, keeps fresh for two weeks.

■

GLYCEMIC INDEX: 54
NUTRIENTS PER SERVING:

CALORIES 220
FAT . . . . 9 g
CARBOHYDRATE . . . . 33 g
FIBER . . . . 4 g

½ *cup butter (1 stick)*

½ *cup honey*

6 *cups old fashioned oats*

1 *cup pecan pieces*

1 *tablespoon cinnamon*

1½ *cups diced dried golden plums (25 halves)*

1. Preheat oven to 350°.

2. Place butter and honey in a large oven-proof lasagne pan and melt in preheated oven (about 2 minutes).

3. In a large mixing bowl, combine the oats, pecans and cinnamon. Add to the melted honey-butter mixture. Combine well, making sure to coat all dry ingredients.

4. Bake for 25 minutes, stirring the mixture every 5 minutes to prevent burning.

5. Remove the granola from the oven and let cool. Add the dried plums. Store in airtight container.

MAKES 18 1/2-CUP SERVINGS

Creamy Oatmeal with Banana and Raisins

A tasty variation on a simple oatmeal dish.

■

GLYCEMIC INDEX: 55
NUTRIENTS PER SERVING:
CALORIES 204
FAT .... 3 g
CARBOHYDRATE .... 38 g
FIBER .... 3 g

1. Place the oats in a saucepan or large microwave bowl. Add sufficient water to cover plus about ⅔ cup of the milk.

2. Bring to a boil and boil 2 minutes or microwave (100% power) for 1 to 2 minutes.

3. Add the banana and cook 1 to 2 minutes more.

4. Add the remaining milk to make a smooth consistency and stir through raisins.

SERVES 2

⅔ cup (2 ozs.) rolled oats

1 cup (8 ozs.) 1% milk, approximately

1 small banana, mashed

1 heaping tablespoon raisins

Fruit 'n' Oat Hotcakes

A moist spicy hotcake, studded with dried ftuit.

■

GLYCEMIC INDEX: 59
NUTRIENTS PER HOTCAKE:

CALORIES........................90
FAT.........................2 g
CARBOHYDRATE ....16 g
FIBER ....2 g

1½ cups (12 ozs.) 1% milk

2 teaspoons honey

1 packet (1 tablespoon) dry
   yeast

⅓ cup (1 oz.) rolled oats

½ cup (2 ozs.) oat bran

⅓ cup (1½ ozs.) currants or
   other dried fruit

½ cup (2½ ozs.) flour

½ teaspoon ground cinna-
   mon

½ teaspoon allspice

fruit spread or jam, to serve

1. Combine the milk and honey in a
   saucepan or microwave bowl and
   warm until lukewarm (about 50 seconds on 100% power in microwave
   oven). Remove from heat and sprinkle
   in the yeast. Mix well with a fork.

2. Combine the rolled oats, bran, currants
   (or other dried fruit) and sifted flour
   and spices in a large bowl. Pour in the
   milk and yeast mixture and stir to
   combine. Let stand in a warm place for
   15 to 30 minutes. Do not stir again.
   Mixture will increase in volume and
   thicken on standing.

3. Heat a nonstick frying pan over moderate heat. Spray with cooking spray or
   lightly grease with butter. Without stirring, take spoonfuls of oat mixture
   from the bowl and drop into the pan.
   Cook until browned underneath, then
   turn and brown on the other side.
   (This will take about 3 to 4 minutes.)

4. Serve hotcakes immediately with fruit
   spread or jam.

MAKES 10 HOTCAKES

Buttermilk Pancakes with Fruit

A light pancake with a lower G.I. than your average pancake. This is achieved by substituting oats or oat bran for some of the flour and including dried fruit.

■

GLYCEMIC INDEX: 56
NUTRIENTS PER PANCAKE:

CALORIES......................118
FAT........................2 g
CARBOHYDRATE...........18 g
FIBER................................2 g

1. Combine the oats and buttermilk in a bowl and let stand 10 minutes.

2. Stir in the dried fruit, flour, sugar, baking soda. Add egg and butter; mix thoroughly.

3. Heat a nonstick frying pan and spray with cooking spray or grease lightly with butter. Pour in about 3 tablespoons of batter, cook over moderate–high heat until bubbly on top and lightly browned underneath. Turn pancake to brown on other side. Repeat with remaining batter.

MAKES ABOUT 10 (SMALL) PANCAKES

1 cup (3 ozs.) 1-minute oats or unprocessed oat bran

2 cups (16 ozs.) buttermilk

½ cup (2¾ ozs.) dried fruit medley, chopped

½ cup (2¾ ozs.) all purpose flour, sifted

2 teaspoons sugar

1 teaspoon baking soda

1 egg, lightly beaten

2 teaspoons butter, melted

Dried fruit medley is a mixture of dried fruit and is available from supermarkets and health food stores.

Mushroom Cheese Omelet

Combined with 100% stoneground whole wheat bread, this omelet offers a hearty and healthy start to any day.

■

GLYCEMIC INDEX: 55
NUTRIENTS PER SERVING:
CALORIES 185
FAT . . . . 12 g
CARBOHYDRATE . . . . 5 g
FIBER . . . . 1 g

3 eggs

1½ tablespoons water

pinch salt and pepper

½ cup onions, diced

½ cup mushrooms, diced

vegetable spray

1 oz. feta cheese, crumbled

½ tablespoon butter

2 slices stoneground whole
    wheat bread

1. Spray a small skillet with vegetable spray and heat on medium flame.

2. Sauté the onions and mushrooms until cooked, about 4 minutes. Place in a small bowl with crumbled feta and set aside.

3. In a small bowl, mix the eggs (preferably at room temperature), water, salt and pepper. Beat until combined. Set aside.

4. Spray the skillet again and heat it over a medium-high flame. Add the butter. When it stops foaming, add the eggs.

5. Shake skillet in a circular motion. As the eggs begin to set, allow the still liquid part to run underneath from time to time by gently pulling the top edges away from the sides of the pan.

6. Continue to shake the skillet. When the omelet is set, add the prepared filling down the center.

7. Lift the skillet at the handle side and, using a spatula, allow the omelet to fold itself in half. Turn off heat.

8. Tip the skillet and allow the omelet to roll onto a warmed plate. Serve immediately with stoneground whole wheat toast.

SERVES 2

Crispy Toast and Tomatoes

You can reduce the fat content of this dish by omitting the butter. The vegetable mixture itself makes a nice accompaniment to eggs.

■

GLYCEMIC INDEX: 54
NUTRIENTS PER SERVING:

CALORIES 165
FAT . . . . 9 g
CARBOHYDRATE . . . . 19 g
FIBER . . . . 2 g

---

1 teaspoon olive oil

1 small leek, washed and finely sliced, approximately ½ cup

5 small mushrooms, sliced, approximately ¾ cup

2 slices low G.I. bread, e.g., 100% stoneground whole wheat

1 tablespoon butter

13½ ozs., about 8 cherry tomatoes, halved

2 teaspoons finely chopped fresh basil or ¼ tsp dried

1 teaspoon finely chopped fresh oregano or ⅛ teaspoon dried

1 teaspoon finely chopped fresh parsley or ⅛ teaspoon dried

freshly ground black pepper

1. Heat the oil in a frying pan, add the leek and mushrooms and cook over medium heat for about 4 to 5 minutes or until tender.

2. Toast the bread and spread with butter.

3. Add the tomatoes and herbs to the leek mixture and cook for 1 to 2 minutes longer, or until heated through. Season to taste with pepper and serve on the toast.

SERVES 2

Soups

TASTY TOMATO AND BASIL SOUP

LENTIL SOUP

MINESTRONE

SPLIT PEA SOUP

■

Tasty Tomato and Basil Soup

*A delicious variation on tomato soup, with a secret
ingredient of sweet potato.*

■

GLYCEMIC INDEX: 54
NUTRIENTS PER SERVING:
CALORIES 105
FAT ....1 g
CARBOHYDRATE ....16 g
FIBER ....2 g

1 teaspoon oil

2 medium orange sweet
potatoes (about 1 lb.),
peeled and chopped

1 large onion (5 ozs.),
coarsely chopped

2 cups (16 ozs.) tomato juice

1 cup (8 ozs.) dry white
wine

2 cups (16 ozs.) prepared
chicken stock

1 bunch fresh basil

salt

freshly ground black pepper

1. Heat the oil in a saucepan, add the
potato and onion and cook over
medium heat for 5 minutes.

2. Add the tomato juice, wine and stock,
simmer, covered, for about 20 minutes,
or until the potato is soft.

3. Add the basil leaves and puree the
soup in a food processor or blender.
Return to the saucepan, add salt and
pepper to taste and reheat.

SERVES 8

Lentil Soup

*A very tasty winter soup, filling and warming—
this makes a meal in itself.*

■

**GLYCEMIC INDEX: 30
NUTRIENTS PER SERVING (SERVING 6):**

CALORIES 166
FAT . . . . .4 g
CARBOHYDRATE . . . . .29 g
FIBER . . . . .8 g

1. Heat the oil in a large saucepan. Add the onion, cover and cook gently for about 10 minutes or until beginning to brown, stirring frequently.

2. Add the garlic, turmeric, curry powder, cumin and chili if desired, and cook, stirring, for 1 minute.

3. Stir in the water, stock, lentils, barley, tomatoes, and salt and pepper to taste. Bring to a boil, cover and simmer about 45 minutes or until the lentils and barley are tender.

4. Serve sprinkled with parsley or coriander.

SERVES 4 TO 6

1 tablespoon oil

1 large onion (5 ozs.), finely chopped

2 cloves garlic, crushed, or 2 teaspoons minced garlic

½ teaspoon turmeric (optional)

2 teaspoons curry powder (optional)

½ teaspoon ground cumin (optional)

1 teaspoon minced chili (optional)

6 cups (48 ozs.) water

1½ cups (12 ozs.) prepared-chicken stock

1 cup (6 ½ ozs.) brown or red lentils

½ cup (3 ½ ozs.) pearled barley

14½ oz. can crushed tomatoes, undrained

salt

freshly ground black pepper

chopped fresh parsley or coriander, to serve

Minestrone

Another delicious stand-alone meal.
Serve with bread and a green salad.

∎

GLYCEMIC INDEX: 37
NUTRIENTS PER SERVING:
CALORIES 145
FAT .... 4 g
CARBOHYDRATE .... 25 g
FIBER .... 5 g

½ cup (3½ ozs.) dried navy beans, or 15 oz. can, rinsed and drained

olive oil, 1 tablespoon

2 medium onions (8 ozs.), chopped

2 cloves garlic, crushed, or 2 teaspoons minced garlic

2 ham bones (about 10 ozs.)

10 cups (2½ quarts) water

5 beef bouillon cubes

3 large carrots (9 ozs.), diced

4 stalks celery (5 ozs.), sliced

2 small zucchini (6½ ozs.), chopped

4 tomatoes (12 ozs.), diced

½ cup (2 ozs.) small macaroni pasta

2 tablespoons chopped fresh parsley

freshly ground black pepper

grated Parmesan cheese, to serve (optional)

1. If using dried navy beans, soak overnight in water to cover by 2 inches.

2. Heat oil in a large heavy-based saucepan. Add the onions and garlic and cook for about 5 minutes or until soft. Add the ham bones, water, bouillon cubes and drained beans (soaked or canned). Bring to a boil and simmer, covered, about 2½ hours or until beans are tender. (Omit the simmering if using canned beans and simply bring to a boil.)

3. Add the carrots, celery, zucchini and tomatoes to the stock. Reduce heat and simmer, covered, 1 hour.

4. Remove the lid, take out the ham bones and add the macaroni to the saucepan. Continue to simmer for about 10 to 15 minutes or until the macaroni is tender.

5. Stir in the parsley and add pepper to taste. Serve with Parmesan cheese, if desired.

SERVES 6

Split Pea Soup

A full flavored favorite that makes an excellent basis for a light meal. Begin this soup a day ahead, allowing the split peas to soak overnight.

■

GLYCEMIC INDEX: 30
NUTRIENTS PER SERVING:

CALORIES 221
FAT . . . . .3 g
CARBOHYDRATE . . . . .41 g
FIBER . . . . .16 g

1. Wash the split peas, place in a large saucepan with the ham bone and water. Bring to a boil.

2. Skim any fat from the top and simmer, covered, for 2 hours.

3. Remove the bones from the soup and trim any meat from them. Return the meat to the soup.

4. Heat the oil in a frying pan, add the onion, carrot and celery and cook for about 10 minutes or until lightly browned. Add the onion mixture to the soup with the bay leaf and thyme. Simmer, covered, for 20 minutes. Remove the bay leaf.

5. Puree the soup in a food processor or blender adding extra water if necessary to make a soup consistency.

6. Add the lemon juice and season to taste with pepper. Reheat if needed before serving.

SERVES 6

2 cups (1 lb.) split peas

1 ham bone (optional)

12 cups (3 quarts) water

1 teaspoon oil

1 medium onion (4 ozs.), finely chopped

1 large carrot (4 ozs.), finely chopped

2 stalks celery (3 ozs.), finely chopped

1 bay leaf

½ teaspoon dried thyme leaves

juice of ½ lemon

freshly ground black pepper

Salads

MUSHROOM AND BULGUR SALAD

PASTA AND BEAN SALAD

RED BEAN SALAD

WHITE BEAN SALAD

TORTELLINI SALAD

LUNCH BOX SALAD

■

Mushroom and Bulgur Salad

This super high fiber salad is a variation on tabouli.
Choose small mushrooms to blend into the salad nicely.

∎

GLYCEMIC INDEX: 48
NUTRIENTS PER SERVING:

CALORIES 176
FAT .... 1 g
CARBOHYDRATE .... 37 g
FIBER .... 9 g

1. Place bulgur and water to cover in a small saucepan. Cover and let simmer until water is absorbed (about 15 minutes).

2. Combine with the remaining ingredients in a bowl. Toss well and serve, warm or chilled.

SERVES 4

1 cup (4.5 ozs.) bulgur (cracked wheat)

1 cup (4.5 ozs.) button mushrooms, canned, drained, sliced

3 scallions, green part only, finely chopped

½ cup (1 oz.) finely chopped fresh parsley

2 tablespoons reduced calorie French dressing

Pasta and Bean Salad

A summer salad full of flavor.
Easy to prepare with canned beans.

■

GLYCEMIC INDEX: 37
NUTRIENTS PER SERVING:

CALORIES 130

FAT . . . . 4 g

CARBOHYDRATE . . . . 19 g

FIBER . . . . 4 g

1 cup (4 ozs.) cooked pasta
(e.g. shells, elbows,
twists)

1 cup (6.5 ozs.) cooked or
canned red kidney beans,
well drained

3 scallions, green part only,
finely chopped

1 tablespoon finely chopped
fresh parsley

DRESSING

1 tablespoon olive oil

1 tablespoon wine vinegar

1 teaspoon Dijon mustard

1 clove garlic, crushed

freshly ground black pepper

1. Combine the pasta, beans, scallions
and parsley in a serving bowl.

2. For the dressing, combine the oil,
vinegar, mustard, garlic and pepper in
a screw-top jar; shake well to combine.

3. Pour the dressing over the pasta mixture and toss well.

SERVES 4

Red Bean Salad

*Serve this delicious salad over crisp
lettuce leaves if desired.*

■

GLYCEMIC INDEX: 52
NUTRIENTS PER SERVING:

CALORIES 131
FAT .... 4 g
CARBOHYDRATE .... 19 g
FIBER .... 7 g

1. Combine the beans, onion and green
   pepper in a bowl.

2. For the dressing, combine all the
   ingredients in a screw-top jar; shake
   well.

3. Add the dressing to the bean mixture
   and toss well. Cover and refrigerate
   overnight to develop flavor.

SERVES 4

*15½ oz. can red kidney
beans, rinsed and drained*

*1 medium white onion (4
ozs.), finely chopped*

*1 medium green pepper (5
ozs.), finely chopped*

DRESSING

*1 tablespoon red wine
vinegar*

1 tablespoon olive oil

pinch salt

1 teaspoon French mustard

*1 clove garlic, crushed, or 1
teaspoon minced garlic*

dash Tabasco sauce

freshly ground black pepper

White Bean Salad

Simple, refreshing and sustaining,
this salad also travels well to work or school.

■

GLYCEMIC INDEX: 36
NUTRIENTS PER SERVING:

CALORIES 109
FAT ....3 g
CARBOHYDRATE ....15 g
FIBER ....4 g

---

19 oz. can cannellini beans

⅓ medium red onion, finely diced

6 sprigs fresh parsley, minced

⅛ teaspoon garlic powder

1 tablespoon olive oil

1. Drain beans, discarding liquid. Place in small serving bowl.

2. Add remaining ingredients. Mix well.

3. May be served cold or at room temperature.

MAKES 5 ½-CUP SERVINGS

Tortellini Salad

*When prepared in advance, the melding of the varied flavors
in this one-dish meal is a palatable delight.*

■

GLYCEMIC INDEX: 50
NUTRIENTS PER SERVING:

CALORIES 277
FAT. . . . . .16 g
CARBOHYDRATE . . . . .20 g
FIBER . . . . .2 g

1. In a small bowl, whisk together dressing ingredients. Set aside.

2. Cook tortellini in boiling water according to package directions.

3. While tortellini are cooking, prepare vegetables: cook broccoli until just tender; spray frying pan with vegetable spray, heat pan and saute peppers and scallions for two minutes, stirring constantly.

4. In a large serving bowl, mix vegetables, ham cubes and pine nuts.

5. Drain cooked tortellini and add them to vegetable mixture.

6. Pour dressing over salad and toss thoroughly. Serve at room temperature or chilled.

MAKES 13 1-CUP SERVINGS

DRESSING:

⅔ *cup olive oil*

⅓ *cup balsamic vinegar*

1 *tablespoon Dijon mustard*

2 *tablespoons fresh parsley, finely chopped*

1 *lb. cheese tortellini*

4 *cups fresh broccoli (2 large stalks), cut up in small pieces*

2 *sweet red peppers, cut in 1-inch julienne strips*

½ *cup scallions, coarsely chopped*

4 *ozs. boiled ham, ½-inch thick slice, cubed*

1 *oz. pine nuts, toasted*

¼ *cup grated cheese*

Lunch Box Salad

A low G.I. salad which makes a tasty alternative to a sandwich. It could be made up the night before, but don't add the dressing until the day of eating.

■

GLYCEMIC INDEX: 52
NUTRIENTS PER SERVING:

CALORIES......................293
FAT.........................7 g
CARBOHYDRATE...........36 g
FIBER......................10 g

about 2 cups shredded lettuce

1 cup (5 ozs.) canned mixed beans, drained

1 cup combined chopped raw vegetables, tomato, mushrooms, onion, cucumber, celery, capsicum, radish, cauliflower, carrot)—in bite-sized pieces

1 slice (1 oz.) ham, chopped into small pieces (optional)

low fat salad dressing

2 tablespoons grated cheddar cheese

1. In a plastic container, place the lettuce. Top with the beans, vegetables and ham if desired.

2. Drizzle dressing over the top and sprinkle over the cheese.

3. Refrigerate until lunch time or enjoy immediately.

SERVES 3

Pastas

CREAMY MUSHROOMS AND PASTA

FETTUCCINE WITH BACON AND MUSHROOM SAUCE

PASTA PRIMAVERA

SPAGHETTI BOLOGNESE

VEGETABLE LASAGNA

■

Creamy Mushrooms and Pasta

*When mushrooms are in season put this dish together
quickly with ingredients from the pantry.*

▪

GLYCEMIC INDEX: 41
NUTRIENTS PER SERVING:

CALORIES 394
FAT . . . . .5 g
CARBOHYDRATE . . . . .68 g
FIBER . . . . .8 g

2 cups (8 ozs.) macaroni or
   other small pasta

2 tablespoons finely
   chopped fresh parsley

2 tablespoons finely grated
   Parmesan cheese

SAUCE

2 teaspoons olive oil

1 medium onion (4 ozs.),
   finely sliced

1 clove garlic, crushed, or
   1 teaspoon minced garlic

1 lb. mushrooms

1 teaspoon paprika

2 teaspoons Dijon mustard

2 tablespoons tomato paste

12 oz. can evaporated skim
   milk

¼ cup (1 oz.) grated low fat
   cheddar cheese

3 scallions, green part only

freshly ground black pepper

1. Add the pasta to a large saucepan of
   boiling water, boil, uncovered, until
   just tender; drain and keep warm.

2. While the pasta is cooking, begin the
   sauce. Heat the oil in a nonstick frying
   pan. Add the onions, garlic and mushrooms, and cook for about 5 minutes
   or until softened.

3. Combine the paprika, mustard, tomato
   paste and milk in a small bowl. Stir
   into the mushroom mixture with the
   cheese and cook stirring frequently
   over low heat for 5 minutes.

4. Add the scallions with pepper to taste.

5. Pour the sauce over the pasta and toss
   gently to combine. Serve sprinkled with
   the parsley and Parmesan cheese.

SERVES 4

*Mushrooms are a good source of niacin
and can be a source of Vitamin B12 if they
are grown on a mixture containing animal
compost.*

Fettuccine with Bacon and Mushroom Sauce

This is a tasty, low fat variation on the traditional creamy sauce of this popular pasta dish. Serve with a tossed green salad.

■

GLYCEMIC INDEX: 41
NUTRIENTS PER SERVING:

CALORIES 340
FAT .... 8 g
CARBOHYDRATE .... 47 g
FIBER .... 4 g

1. Cut the bacon into short, thin slices. Cook in a nonstick frying pan until browned. Meanwhile, add the fettuccine to a large saucepan of boiling water, boil, uncovered, until just tender; drain.

2. Add the mushrooms and oil to the frying pan with the bacon, cook for 2 minutes.

3. Stir in the mustard and wine and cook 3 minutes. Reduce the heat, add the cheese and stir until melted.

4. Add the blended cornstarch and water, stir over low heat until the mixture becomes quite thick.

5. Remove from the heat and cool slightly. Gradually add the buttermilk and pepper, stirring until well combined. Do not heat or the sauce may curdle.

6. Serve the sauce immediately over the fettuccine. Serve with Parmesan cheese, if desired.

SERVES 4

5 ozs. Canadian bacon, 5.5 slices

8 ozs. fettuccine pasta

2.5 ozs. small mushrooms, sliced

1 tablespoon oil

1 teaspoon whole grain mustard

2 tablespoons red or white wine (optional)

¼ cup (1 oz.) grated low-fat cheddar cheese

2 teaspoons cornstarch

2 tablespoons water

½ cup (4 ozs.) buttermilk

freshly ground black pepper

grated Parmesan cheese, to serve (optional)

Pasta Primavera

*A simple, light pasta dish that can be on
the plate in about 15 minutes.*

∎

GLYCEMIC INDEX: 42
NUTRIENTS PER SERVING:

CALORIES 230
FAT .... 8 g
CARBOHYDRATE .... 33 g
FIBER .... 6 g

---

*4 ozs. uncooked spaghetti or
other pasta*

1 tablespoon of olive oil

*2 medium zucchini (8 ozs.),
cut in thin diagonal slices*

*1 cup (8 ozs.) mushrooms,
thinly sliced*

*1 clove garlic, crushed
or 1 tablespoon minced
garlic*

*3½ ozs. (about 8)
cherry tomatoes, halved*

*1 tablespoon grated
Parmesan cheese*

fresh basil leaves (optional)

1. Cook the spaghetti in a large saucepan
   of boiling water, according to package
   directions.

2. Meanwhile, heat the olive oil in a large
   frying pan. Add the zucchini, mushrooms and garlic, saute lightly for 5
   minutes.

3. Drain the spaghetti and return to the
   saucepan. Add the vegetables and stir
   through. Top with grated Parmesan
   and strips of fresh basil leaves if
   desired. Serve hot or warm.

SERVES 3

Spaghetti Bolognese

To keep the fat content down, use a minimum amount of oil and the leanest possible ground beef.

■

GLYCEMIC INDEX: 43
NUTRIENTS PER SERVING:

CALORIES 578
FAT .... 14 g
CARBOHYDRATE .... 72 g
FIBER 7

1. Heat the oil in a saucepan or frying pan, add the onion, carrot, celery, and garlic and cook for about 10 minutes, or until the onion is very soft, stirring frequently. Cover if drying out too much. Add bacon bits.

2. Increase the heat and add the beef. Cook for about 5 minutes, stirring constantly until the beef is crumbly and browned.

3. Add the tomato paste, tomatoes, wine and stock. Bring to a boil. Add the oregano, pepper, bay leaf and nutmeg and stir thoroughly. Cover and simmer for 1 hour, stirring frequently to prevent sticking. Remove bay leaf.

4. Meanwhile, add the spaghetti to a large saucepan of boiling water and boil, uncovered, until just tender, 10–12 minutes; drain.

5. Serve the beef ragu over the spaghetti. Sprinkle with parsley and serve with Parmesan cheese, if desired.

SERVES 4

1 tablespoon olive oil

1 very small onion (2½ ozs.), finely chopped

1 carrot (3 ozs.), grated

2 stalks celery (2 ozs.), sliced

2 cloves garlic, crushed, or 2 teaspoons minced garlic

1 oz. bacon bits

10 ozs. lean ground beef

2 tablespoons tomato paste

14 oz. can tomatoes, undrained and mashed

¼ cup (2 ozs.) dry red wine

¼ cup (2 ozs.) beef stock

¼ teaspoon dried oregano leaves

freshly ground black pepper

1 bay leaf

2 pinches grated nutmeg

12 ozs. spaghetti

chopped fresh parsley, to serve (optional)

grated Parmesan cheese

Vegetable Lasagna

*A tasty, moist lasagna packed with goodies
from beans to pasta.*

■

GLYCEMIC INDEX: 45
NUTRIENTS PER SERVING:

CALORIES 347
FAT. . . . . .10 g
CARBOHYDRATE . . . . .54 g
FIBER . . . . .9 g

1 10 oz. bag spinach,
  washed and stems
  removed

12 instant lasagna sheets

2 tablespoons (⅔ oz.)
  grated Parmesan cheese
  or low fat cheddar cheese

VEGETABLE SAUCE

2 teaspoons olive oil

2 medium onions (8 ozs.),
  chopped

2 cloves garlic, crushed, or
  2 teaspoons minced garlic

8 ozs. mushrooms, sliced

1 small green pepper
  (3.5 ozs.), chopped

½ cup tomato paste

15 oz. can white beans,
  rinsed and drained

1. Blanch or lightly steam the spinach
   until just wilted; drain well.

2. For the vegetable sauce, heat the oil in
   a nonstick frying pan. Add the onions
   and garlic and cook for about 5 minutes or until soft. Add the mushrooms
   and green pepper and cook 3 minutes,
   stirring occasionally. Add the tomato
   paste, beans, tomatoes and herbs.
   Bring to a boil and simmer, partly covered, for 15 to 20 minutes.

3. Meanwhile, for the cheese sauce, melt
   the butter in a saucepan or in a
   microwave bowl. Stir in the flour and
   cook 1 minute, stirring (for 30 seconds
   100% power, in microwave). Remove
   from the heat. Gradually add the milk,
   stirring until smooth. Stir over medium
   heat until the sauce boils and thickens,
   or in microwave (100% power) until
   boiling, stirring occasionally. Remove
   from the heat, stir in the cheese, nutmeg and pepper.

4. To assemble, pour half the vegetable
   sauce over the base of a lasagna dish,
   rectangular pan or ovenproof dish

14.5 oz. can tomatoes,
    undrained, crushed

1 teaspoon Italian seasoning

CHEESE SAUCE

4 teaspoons butter

1 tablespoon all purpose flour

1½ cups (12 ozs.) 1% milk

½ cup (2 ozs.) grated cheese

pinch ground nutmeg

(about 6 inch by 11 inch). Cover with a layer of lasagna sheets, then half the spinach. Spread a thin layer of cheese sauce over the spinach. Top with the remaining vegetable sauce and remaining spinach. Place over a layer of lasagna sheets and finish with the remaining cheese sauce. Sprinkle with Parmesan or cheddar cheese.

5. Cover with aluminum foil and bake in a moderate oven 350° for 40 minutes. Remove foil and bake for 30 minutes or until the top is beginning to brown.

SERVES 6

Dipping the lasagna sheets briefly in hot water before use helps to soften them prior to cooking.

Main Dishes

CHICKEN AND BASMATI RICE PILAF

CURRY RICE WITH CHICKEN SAUCE

BEEF AND LENTIL PATTIES

"HOT" FAJITA POCKETS

VEGETABLE VEAL STIR-FRY

MEGA-VEG MEAT LOAF

FISH AND CHILI BEANS

GREEN CHEESE PIE

WINTER CHILI HOTPOT

FRIED BASMATI RICE

MEDITERRANEAN RICE AND BEANS

SPINACH CHEESE BAKE

MOROCCAN BURGERS

SPICY PILAF WITH CHICKPEAS

SWEET 'N' SPICY CHICKEN STIR FRY

QUICK AND EASY CHILI

■

Chicken and Basmati Rice Pilaf

This is a flavorsome one-pot meal, best served with a salad. High in carbohydrate, it's especially good for active people.

■

GLYCEMIC INDEX: 59
NUTRIENTS PER SERVING:

CALORIES 612

FAT .... 13 g

CARBOHYDRATE .... 84 g

FIBER .... 3 g

1. Heat the oil in a medium to large saucepan, add the chicken and cook, stirring, over medium heat for about 10 minutes or until beginning to brown. Transfer to a plate.

2. Melt the butter in the same pan, add the onion and pepper and cook for about 5 minutes or until soft.

3. Add the rosemary and cook 3 minutes or until the onion is lightly browned. Return the chicken to the pan, add the rice and stir.

4. Pour the cold stock over the chicken and rice mixture and bring to a boil. Cover with a tight-fitting lid and simmer gently for 20 minutes or until the rice is tender and the liquid is absorbed.

SERVES 2 AS A MAIN COURSE

1 teaspoon olive oil

2 chicken cutlets (about 4 ozs.), skinned and sliced

2 teaspoons butter

1 large (5 ozs.) purple Spanish onion, sliced

½ medium red pepper (2 ½ ozs.), sliced

½ teaspoon dried rosemary leaves

1 cup (6½ ozs.) Basmati rice

2 cups (16 ozs.) prepared chicken stock

Curry Rice with Chicken Sauce

*This is a very high carbohydrate dish and a
good choice for all sports people.*

▪

GLYCEMIC INDEX: 58
NUTRIENTS PER SERVING:
CALORIES......................482
FAT........................10 g
CARBOHYDRATE ....64 g
FIBER ....3 g

2 boned chicken breasts (12 ozs.), skin removed

1 tablespoon oil

1 onion (5 ozs.), finely chopped

2 stalks celery (2½ ozs.), sliced

1 medium carrot (4 ozs.), grated

6 sprigs fresh parsley, finely chopped

½ cup (4 ozs.) dry white wine

2 teaspoons tomato paste

½ cup (4 ozs.) chicken stock

freshly ground black pepper

1 bay leaf

2 tablespoons (⅔ oz.) grated Parmesan cheese, to serve

CURRY RICE

3 cups (24 ozs.) water

1½ cups (10 ozs.) long grain rice

1 teaspoon butter

1 teaspoon curry powder

1. Cut the chicken into ½ inch cubes.

2. Heat the oil in a saucepan or nonstick frying pan. Add the vegetables and parsley, and cook gently for 10 minutes, stirring frequently.

3. Add the chicken and cook, stirring, for 4 to 5 minutes. Add the wine and boil quickly until it evaporates. Stir in the combined tomato paste and stock. Season with pepper and add the bay leaf. Bring to a boil, reduce the heat and simmer gently for 15 minutes. Remove the bay leaf.

4. Meanwhile, cook the rice. Bring the water to a boil in a saucepan, add the rice and simmer, covered, for about 18 to 20 minutes or until all the water is absorbed. Drain and rinse well under hot water. Return to the saucepan, add the butter and curry powder, stir until combined.

5. Place the rice into a warmed serving dish, top with the chicken sauce and sprinkle with the Parmesan cheese.

SERVES 4

Beef and Lentil Patties

Serve these succulent patties hot with vegetables or
salad and mustard or ketchup.

■

GLYCEMIC INDEX: 34
NUTRIENTS PER PATTY:
CALORIES........................48
FAT........................2 g
CARBOHYDRATE ....4 g
FIBER 1

1. Cook the lentils in a saucepan of boiling water for about 20 minutes or until soft; drain well.

2. Combine the lentils with the beef, onion, pepper, garlic, herbs, sauce, egg and pepper in a bowl; mix well.

3. Add enough oat bran to form a burger consistency. Shape the mixture into 24 small patties and place on a lightly greased baking tray.

4. Bake in a hot oven (400°) for about 40 minutes, or until cooked through, turning halfway through cooking time. Alternatively, cook the patties in a nonstick frying pan over medium-high heat or until browned and cooked through.

MAKES 24 SMALL PATTIES

½ cup (3 ozs.) brown or red lentils

12 ozs. lean ground beef

1 medium onion (4 ozs.), finely chopped

½ small pepper (2 ozs.), finely chopped

1 clove garlic, crushed, or 1 teaspoon minced garlic

2 teaspoons dried mixed herbs

⅓ cup (3 ozs.) tomato sauce

1 egg, lightly beaten

freshly ground black pepper

about ½ cup (2½ ozs.) unprocessed oat bran

Reheat the leftovers and serve sandwiched in pita bread with ketchup, tomato, cucmber, grated carrot and lettuce.

"Hot" Fajita Pockets

*Some like it hot—and here it is! The flavorful hot peppers,
however, can be reduced or eliminated to suit individual tastes.*

■

GLYCEMIC INDEX: 57
NUTRIENTS PER SERVING:

CALORIES 299

FAT . . . . 8 g

CARBOHYDRATE . . . . 37 g

FIBER . . . . 3 g

MARINADE:

1 tablespoon oil

2 tablespoons soy sauce

*2 tablespoons fresh ginger,
grated or 1 teaspoon
ground*

2 tablespoons minced garlic

*1 lb. lean beef, eye round or
London broil*

8 large (2 ozs.) corn tortillas

vegetable spray

*2 large onions, coarsely
chopped*

8 ozs. mushrooms, slices

½ cup kidney beans, drained

*½ teaspoon crushed hot red
pepper*

1. In a medium bowl, whisk together marinade ingredients. Set aside.

2. Wash and pat dry beef with paper towels. Cut into small thin strips, 1 inch x ¼ inch.

3. Marinate beef at least 30 minutes or overnight.

4. Warm tortillas in 200° oven for 10 minutes, placing paper towels between layers while stacking them on a baking sheet. Cover top layer.

5. Spray wok or large frying pan with vegetable spray.

6. Sauté onions in heated pan for 3 minutes, stirring frequently. Add mushrooms and kidney beans and continue sauteing for three minutes.

7. Add beef strips and hot pepper and sauté for another 3 minutes. Continue to stir.

8. Remove warmed tortillas one at a time. Place ⅛ of beef mixture in center of tor

tilla and fold in 4 sides toward middle to form a square pocket. Place on a baking sheet, folded side down.

9. Repeat with remaining tortillas and beef mixture.

10. Return folded pockets to heated oven for 15 minutes. Serve immediately.

MAKES 8 1-POCKET SERVINGS

Vegetable Veal Stir-Fry

*Loaded with vegetables, this high carbohydrate dish
is a very low fat main meal.*

■

GLYCEMIC INDEX: 44
NUTRIENTS PER SERVING:

CALORIES 334
FAT . . . . 3 g
CARBOHYDRATE . . . . 54 g
FIBER . . . . 10 g

12 ozs. spaghetti pasta

2 teaspoons oil

1 medium onion (4 ozs.),
chopped

1 tablespoon grated fresh
ginger or 1 tablespoon
minced ginger

1 clove garlic, crushed, or
1 teaspoon minced garlic

6 ozs. veal cutlets, cut into
thin strips

2 stalks celery (2½ ozs.),
sliced

1 small yellow pepper (3
ozs.), chopped

1 medium red pepper (5
ozs.), chopped

6 ozs. cauliflower, cut into
florets

1 large carrot (5 ozs.),
chopped

6 ozs. broccoli, chopped

1. Add the spaghetti to a large saucepan
of boiling water, boil, uncovered, until
just tender; drain and keep warm.

2. Heat the oil in a wok or large nonstick
frying pan. Add the onion, ginger, garlic and veal. Stir-fry over medium heat
for about 3 to 5 minutes or until the
veal is almost cooked.

3. Add the remaining vegetables and stir-
fry until just tender, sprinkling in a
little water if necessary.

4. Stir in the blended sauce(s), cornstarch
and water. Stir until the mixture boils
and thickens.

5. Add the spaghetti; stir until heated
through. Serve immediately.

SERVES 6

12 ozs. portobello mush-
rooms, sliced

1 bunch fresh asparagus,
chopped

1 tablespoon salt-reduced
soy sauce

¼ cup black bean sauce

1½ tablespoons cornstarch

⅔ cup (5½ ozs.) water

Almost any selection of colorful vegetables
can be used.

Mega-Veg Meat Loaf

A very moist and tender meat loaf. By adding plenty of vegetables to the meat, the fat content of the whole dish is reduced.

■

GLYCEMIC INDEX: 62
NUTRIENTS PER SERVING:
CALORIES 299
FAT . . . . 12 g
CARBOHYDRATE . . . . 21 g
FIBER 4

1 teaspoon oil

1 medium onion (4 ozs.), finely chopped

1 clove garlic, crushed, or 1 teaspoon minced garlic

3 ozs. small mushrooms, finely sliced

1 lb. lean ground beef

1 cup (3 ozs.) rolled oats

1 small zucchini (3 ozs.), grated

1 medium carrot (4 ozs.), grated

½ cup (2½ ozs.) green peas

2 tablespoons tomato sauce

1 teaspoon Worcestershire sauce

1 egg, lightly beaten

1 teaspoon dried basil leaves

½ teaspoon dried oregano leaves

½ teaspoon dried thyme leaves

¼ cup finely chopped fresh parsley

1. Heat the oil in a nonstick frying pan, add the onion, garlic and mushrooms and cook for about 5 minutes or until just soft; cool.

2. Combine the remaining ingredients in a large bowl. Add the onion mixture and mix well.

3. Press the mixture into a lightly greased loaf pan (about 9 x 5 x 2¾ inches). Cover with foil.

4. Bake in a hot oven (400°) for about 1 hour or until done.

SERVES 6

Fish and Chili Beans

Serve this dish alongside Basmati rice.

■

GLYCEMIC INDEX: 27
NUTRIENTS PER SERVING:

CALORIES 223
FAT .... 5 g
CARBOHYDRATE .... 23 g
FIBER 6

1. Heat the oil in a nonstick frying pan or saucepan. Add the celery, onion and garlic and cook for about 5 minutes or until softened. Add the tomatoes, beans and chili powder. Simmer, uncovered, for 10 minutes.

2. Meanwhile, heat the wine in a medium saucepan over moderate heat. Add the fish and poach gently for about 3 to 4 minutes or until just cooked through.

3. Combine the undrained fish with the tomato and bean mixture. Add the parsley with pepper to taste. Serve immediately.

SERVES 4

2 teaspoons oil

2 stalks celery (2½ ozs.), finely diced

1 medium onion (4 ozs.), finely chopped

1 clove garlic, crushed, or 1 teaspoon minced garlic

14½ oz. can tomatoes, crushed and undrained

15 oz. can butter beans, well drained

⅓ teaspoon chili powder

½ cup (4 ozs.) dry white wine

4 boneless white fish fillets (1 lb.), cut into cubes

2 tablespoons chopped fresh parsley

freshly ground black pepper

Green Cheese Pie

A cheese and egg dish incorporating rice.
Serve with a tossed salad.

▪

GLYCEMIC INDEX: 51
NUTRIENTS PER SERVING:

CALORIES 207
FAT .... 4 g
CARBOHYDRATE .... 28 g
FIBER .... 3 g

½ cup (3 ozs.) Basmati rice

1 cup (1½ ozs.) chopped fresh parsley

1 cup (4 ozs.) grated low-fat cheddar cheese

1 large (5 ozs.) onion, finely chopped

½ cup (4 ozs.) creamed corn

½ cup (4 ozs.) corn kernels

1 large zucchini (6 ozs.), grated

1 oz. mushrooms, finely chopped

3 eggs

2 cups (16 ozs.) skim milk

¼ teaspoon ground nutmeg

1 teaspoon ground cumin

1 egg white, lightly beaten

1. Add the rice to a saucepan of boiling water, boil, uncovered, for about 12 minutes or until just tender; drain.

2. Combine the rice, parsley, half the cheese, onion, creamed corn, corn kernels, zucchini and mushrooms in a bowl and spoon into a greased 9 inch pie dish.

3. Whisk the eggs, milk, nutmeg and cumin in a bowl. Fold in the lightly beaten egg white and pour evenly over the rice mixture. Sprinkle the remaining cheese on top.

4. Bake in a moderate oven (350°) for about 1 hour or until set in the center.

SERVES 6

Winter Chili Hotpot

A tasty one-pot meal that can be prepared in around 30 minutes using canned beans. You could serve it with a dinner roll and side salad.

■

GLYCEMIC INDEX: 38
NUTRIENTS PER SERVING (SERVING 6):

CALORIES	234
FAT	2 g
CARBOHYDRATE	47 g
FIBER	12 g

1. If using dried beans, soak overnight in water to cover. Drain. Bring the water to a boil in a large saucepan, add the beans and bay leaf. Boil rapidly for 15 minutes, then reduce heat and simmer for 40 minutes. Drain and set aside. Omit this step if using canned beans.

2. Heat the oil in a nonstick frying pan, add the onion and garlic and cook for about 5 minutes or until soft.

3. Add the celery, squash or zucchini and mushrooms, cook, stirring, for 5 minutes. Stir in the beans (cooked or canned), tomatoes, chili, tomato paste and stock, and bring to the boil.

4. Add the pasta, reduce heat and simmer for about 20 minutes or until the pasta is tender. Add pepper to taste and serve sprinkled with parsley.

SERVES 4 TO 6

1 cup (6 ozs.) dried red kidney beans or 15½ oz. can kidney beans, rinsed and drained

5 cups (1¼ quarts) water

1 bay leaf

1 teaspoon oil

1 onion, finely chopped

2 cloves garlic, crushed or 2 teaspoons minced garlic

4 stalks celery (5 ozs.), sliced

2 squash or 2 small zucchini (6 ozs.), sliced

8 ozs. button mushrooms

28 oz. can tomatoes, undrained and chopped

1 teaspoon minced chili or ⅓ teaspoon chili powder

2 tablespoons tomato paste

1½ cups (12 ozs.) prepared vegetable stock

1¼ cups (8 ozs.) small macaroni pasta

freshly ground black pepper

chopped fresh parsley, to serve

Fried Basmati Rice

Serve as a light meal or an accompaniment to a stir-fry. If you can't find Basmati, try another long grain rice.

■

GLYCEMIC INDEX: 56
NUTRIENTS PER SERVING (SERVING 6):

CALORIES 434
FAT.........................,........14 g
CARBOHYDRATE ....65 g
FIBER ....5 g

2 cups (13 ozs.) Basmati rice

2 tablespoons oil

3 large eggs, lightly beaten

2 large slices ham, 8 ozs., chopped

1 teaspoon minced ginger

1 cup (5 ozs.) cooked green peas

9 oz. can corn kernels, drained

4 scallions, sliced

1½ tablespoons oyster sauce

2 teaspoons soy sauce

1 tablespoon chicken stock

½ teaspoon sesame oil

1. Place the rice into a saucepan with enough water to cover by 1 inch. Bring to a boil, cover with a tight-fitting lid and simmer very gently for 20 minutes. Remove from heat, stir with a fork to separate the grains and set aside to cool.

2. Heat half the oil in a frying pan, add the eggs and cook over medium heat, stirring with a fork, for 2 to 3 minutes or until set. Remove from pan and cool.

3. Heat the remaining oil in the same pan and stir-fry the ham.

4. Add the rice to the frying pan. Stir in the ginger, peas, corn and scallions and toss gently until heated through. Add the combined sauces, stock and sesame oil and stir to coat the rice thoroughly.

5. Stir in the egg and serve immediately.

SERVES 4 TO 6 AS A LIGHT MAIN COURSE

Mediterranean Rice and Beans

Here is a nutrient powerhouse.
A tossed salad and fruited yogurt are worthy complements.

∎

GLYCEMIC INDEX: 56
NUTRIENTS PER SERVING:

CALORIES 323
FAT .... 6 g
CARBOHYDRATE .... 52 g
FIBER .... 5 g

1. Cook bacon strips until crisp, drain on paper towels and crumble. Set aside.

2. Pour oil in a large pot and heat over medium flame for 20 seconds.

3. Add chopped vegetables and sauté for 5 minutes, stirring frequently.

4. Add rice and mix well. Add wine and allow it to evaporate. Reduce flame.

5. Gradually add broth, ½ cup at a time. Stir carefully and frequently to prevent sticking. Add bacon. Cook slowly for 10 minutes.

6. Add the *undrained* kidney beans. Continue to cook and stir for approximately 5 minutes.

7. Remove rice from heat; stir in parsley. Serve hot.

YIELD: 8 1-CUP SERVINGS

10 *strips center cut bacon*

1 *tablespoon olive oil*

2 *stalks celery, chopped*

1 *medium carrot, chopped*

1 *small onion, chopped*

¼ *cup sun dried tomatoes, chopped*

2 *cups long grain rice*

½ *cup red wine*

3½ *cups broth, beef or vegetable*

1 *can (15 ½ ozs.) red kidney beans*

2 *tablespoons fresh parsley, chopped*

Spinach Cheese Bake

Because of the large quantity of spinach, this dish is a four-star contributor of Vitamin A, folate, calcium and fiber.

■

GLYCEMIC INDEX: 69
NUTRIENTS PER SERVING:
CALORIES 216
FAT .... 7 g
CARBOHYDRATE .... 8 g
FIBER .... 4 g

2 10-oz. bags fresh spinach

3 cups part skim ricotta cheese

1 cup bread crumbs

½ cup grated cheese

1 cup egg substitute

1. Preheat oven to 350°.

2. Thoroughly wash spinach and cook it for 5 minutes in a small amount of water. When cooked, drain spinach and press out excess water.

3. In a bowl, combine spinach, ricotta, ¾ cup bread crumbs, grated cheese and egg substitute.

4. Spray the bottom and sides of a 9 inch square baking pan with vegetable spray. Coat with 2 tablespoons of bread crumbs.

5. Evenly spread spinach mixture in pan. Sprinkle top with remaining bread crumbs.

6. Bake for 45-50 minutes until top is lightly browned. Wait about 10 minutes before cutting into 9 squares.

MAKES 9 3-INCH SQUARES

Moroccan Burgers

■

GLYCEMIC INDEX: 55
NUTRIENTS PER SERVING:

CALORIES 497

FAT ....15 g

CARBOHYDRATE ....57 g

FIBER ....10 g

1. Wrap the pita bread in foil and heat in the oven for 15 minutes.

2. Meanwhile, combine ground beef, bulgur, seasoning, onion and egg in a bowl. Shape mixture into 8 patties.

3. Heat a nonstick pan with cooking spray and cook patties about 7 minutes each side.

4. Combine tomato and mint with olive oil and vinegar in a bowl and serve with the patties and lettuce on the pita bread.

SERVES 4

4 2-oz. *pita loaves*

12 ozs. *lean ground beef*

½ cup (3 ozs.) *bulgur (cracked wheat)*

1 teaspoon *ground cumin*

½ teaspoon *paprika*

½ teaspoon *garlic powder*

⅛ teaspoon *cayenne*

1 medium (4 oz.) *white onion, very finely chopped*

1 egg, *lightly beaten*

1 teaspoon *olive oil*

1 teaspoon *red wine vinegar*

3 medium *tomatoes, diced*

1 tablespoon *coarsely chopped fresh mint or 1 teaspoon dried*

lettuce

Spicy Pilaf with Chickpeas

A meatless rice dish which serves 3–4 for a light meal

•

GLYCEMIC INDEX: 55

NUTRIENTS PER SERVING (SERVING 4):

CALORIES 236

FAT . . . . 8 g

CARBOHYDRATE . . . . 32 g

FIBER . . . . 4 g

1 teaspoon butter

2 teaspoons olive oil

1 medium (5 ozs.) onion, peeled and finely diced

1 clove garlic, crushed

5 ozs. button mushrooms, quartered or halved

⅔ cup Basmati rice

1 teaspoon garam masala*

1 bay leaf

10 oz. can chickpeas (drained)

1½ cups (12 ozs.) chicken stock

1 tablespoon slivered almonds, toasted

*Note: garam masala is an Indian mixture of spices containing cinnamon, bay leaves, cumin seeds, coriander seeds, cardamon seeds, black pepper corns, dried jalapeno, cloves and nutmeg; you can find it in specialty or health food stores

1. Heat butter and oil in a medium sized frying pan over medium heat. Add the onion, cover and cook 3 minutes, stirring occasionally. Add mushrooms and garlic and cook, uncovered a further 5 minutes, stirring occasionally.

2. Add the rice and spice, stirring to combine until aromatic. Add the chickpeas, bay leaf and pour over stock. Bring to the boil. Reduce heat to very low. Cover with a tight-fitting lid and simmer (without lifting the lid) for at least 12 minutes or until rice is tender and all liquid has been absorbed.

3. Sprinkle with toasted almonds and serve with a salad.

SERVES 3 TO 4

Slivered almonds can be easily toasted by placing in a dry pan over medium heat. Once the pan gets hot, toss the almonds around to toast them. This will take no more than a minute. Don't leave unattended because the almonds toast rapidly.

Sweet 'n' Spicy Chicken Stir-Fry

■

GLYCEMIC INDEX: 54
NUTRIENTS PER SERVING:

CALORIES 504
FAT........................13 g
CARBOHYDRATE ....50 g
FIBER ....7 g

1. Cook pasta according to manufacturer's directions. Drain and set aside.

2. Parboil the squash (2 minutes in microwave).

3. Stir fry the strips of chicken in batches in a lightly oiled wok or fry pan. Remove each batch once done and set aside on a plate.

4. Once all the chicken is done, heat the oil in the pan and stir-fry the onion and eggplant a few minutes. Add the pepper strips, cook for 2 minutes. Then add the crushed garlic and diced squash.

5. Return the chicken to the pan, then add the combined chili sauce, honey and soy sauce, all at once. Stir-fry 30 seconds. Toss through the cooked noodles and serve.

SERVES 2

½ inch thick slice of butternut squash (5 ozs.), cut into cubes

2 ozs. angel hair (capellini) pasta

10 ozs. chicken tenders

2 teaspoons oil

½ medium (2½ ozs.) onion, thinly sliced

½ small (6 ozs.) eggplant, cut into ½ inch dices

½ (6 ozs.) small red pepper, cut into narrow strips

1 large clove of garlic or a heaped teaspoon minced garlic

1 tablespoon Thai sweet chili sauce

2 teaspoons honey

2 teaspoons soy sauce

Quick and Easy Chili

This vegetarian chili can be used in lots of dishes—serve it in corn tortillas or taco shells for a Mexican meal, layer it in a vegetable lasagna, or serve it with pasta or rice.

■

GLYCEMIC INDEX: 58
NUTRIENTS PER SERVING:

CALORIES 147

FAT .... 1 g

CARBOHYDRATE .... 25 g

FIBER .... 9 g

1 onion, chopped

2 garlic cloves, crushed

1 can (14½ ozs.) crushed tomatoes

1 small can (5 ozs.) tomato puree

3 teaspoons chili paste or powder

1 teaspoon red or white wine vinegar

pinch dried oregano

pinch dried basil

1 can (15½ ozs.) red kidney beans, drained

1. Coat a large nonstick skillet with cooking spray and heat over medium heat. Add the onions, cover and cook until soft, add garlic as onions soften.

2. Add the remaining ingredients, and simmer, covered, for 30 minutes, stirring occasionally.

SERVES 4

Side Dishes

OVEN ROASTED VEGETABLE MEDLEY

COUSCOUS TRICOLORE

SPICY NOODLES

BAKED BARLEY

SWEET POTATO AND CORN FRITTERS

HOT POTATO SALAD

■

Oven Roasted Vegetable Medley

*This is an easy-to-do recipe that some cooks may want to double.
Leftovers easily fill pita pockets for a next-day lunch.*

■

GLYCEMIC INDEX: 55
NUTRIENTS PER SERVING:

CALORIES.........................90
FAT...........................4 g
CARBOHYDRATE..............9 g
FIBER.......................6 g

3 medium carrots, peeled
and cut into 1-inch slices

4 ozs. mushrooms, halved

1 large yellow squash, cut
into large julienne strips

6 ozs. Brussel sprouts

4 ozs. sweet potato, cut into
1-inch slices

1 tablespoon olive oil

¼ teaspoon thyme, dried

salt and pepper to taste

1½ cups vegetable broth

1. Preheat oven to 425°

2. Wash and cut all the vegetables and
place in a medium bowl. Toss vegetables with olive oil, salt, pepper and
thyme.

3. Place the vegetables in an oblong roast-
ing pan. Pour in the broth.

4. Roast 30–35 minutes until the vegetables are tender. Stir frequently. Serve
hot.

MAKES 4 1-CUP SERVINGS

Couscous Tricolore

Accompany this user-friendly grain with beans,
tofu or grilled vegetables.

■

GLYCEMIC INDEX: 62
NUTRIENTS PER SERVING:

CALORIES 174
FAT ....2 g
CARBOHYDRATE ....30 g
FIBER ....2 g

1. Bring broth to boil. Add couscous and stir.

2. Return liquid to boil, then *simmer* for 2 minutes. Remove from heat and leave covered for 5 minutes.

3. Add oil and mix well.

4. Add remaining ingredients, combining well. Serve.

MAKES 6 ½-CUP SERVINGS

1 cup couscous, uncooked

1½ cups broth, vegetable or chicken

1 teaspoon oil

1 medium tomato, seeded and diced

¼ cup crumbled feta

8 olives, pitted and chopped

Spicy Noodles

Serve these extra spicy noodles alongside something plain or as part of a stir-fry with vegetables.

■

GLYCEMIC INDEX: 34
NUTRIENTS PER SERVING:

CALORIES 289
FAT .... 6 g
CARBOHYDRATE .... 45 g
FIBER .... 4 g

8 ozs. dried thin egg noodles

2 teaspoons oil

2 cloves garlic, crushed, or
   2 teaspoons minced garlic

1 teaspoon minced ginger

1 teaspoon minced chili

6 scallions, sliced

1 tablespoon smooth
   peanut butter

2 tablespoons soy sauce

1 cup (8 ozs.) prepared
   chicken stock

1. Boil the noodles uncovered, for about 5 minutes or until just tender.

2. While the noodles are cooking, heat the oil in a nonstick frying pan, add the garlic, ginger, chili and scallions and stir-fry for 1 minute. Remove from the heat.

3. Stir in the peanut butter and soy sauce and gradually add the stock, stirring until smooth. Stir over heat until simmering, and simmer for 2 minutes.

4. Drain the noodles and add to the spicy sauce, stirring to coat. Serve immediately.

SERVES 4

Baked Barley

*Try barley as a terrific low G.I. accompaniment to a main meal.
Prepared this way it is very tasty but does take some time to cook.*

■

GLYCEMIC INDEX: 25
NUTRIENTS PER SERVING:

CALORIES 179
FAT .... 7 g
CARBOHYDRATE .... 45 g
FIBER .... 5 g

1. Toss the peppers and oil together in a large casserole dish. Bake in a hot oven (400°) for 30 minutes.

2. Add the barley and stir until coated with oil. Add the stock, cover tightly and bake for about 1 hour or until all the stock is absorbed and the barley is tender—add extra stock if necessary.

3. Do not stir the mixture once cooked. Cover and keep warm until ready to serve. Serve with Parmesan cheese, if desired.

SERVES 4

2 *large red peppers*
    (6½ ozs.), cut into strips

1 *tablespoon olive oil*

1 *cup (6½ ozs.) pearled*
    barley

3 *cups (24 ozs.) prepared*
    chicken stock

½ *cup (2 ozs.) grated*
    Parmesan or low fat
    cheddar cheese (optional)

Sweet Potato and Corn Fritters

*A different and easy way to serve potato. The sweet potato gives
the fritters a distinctive flavor and lowers the GI factor.*

•

GLYCEMIC INDEX: 56
NUTRIENTS PER FRITTER: SERVING:

CALORIES 134
FAT . . . . 2 g
CARBOHYDRATE . . . . 26 g
FIBER . . . . 3 g

1 medium sweet potato
(12 ozs.), peeled and
coarsely chopped

2 small potatoes (6 ozs.),
peeled and coarsely
chopped

1 medium onion (4 ozs.),
finely chopped

1 egg, lightly beaten

7 oz. can corn kernels
(drained)

freshly ground black pepper

½ cup (1½ ozs.) rolled oats

2 tablespoons self-rising
flour

extra flour

1 teaspoon oil

1. Combine the potatoes and onion and
steam or microwave together until the
potatoes are tender.

2. Mash the potatoes and onion with the
egg. Add the corn, pepper to taste,
rolled oats and self-rising flour; mix
until well combined.

3. Refrigerate the mixture for 30 minutes
or until completely cooled (this makes
it much easier to shape).

4. Shape the mixture into 8 rounds, coat-
ing gently with extra flour.

5. Heat 1 teaspoon of oil in a nonstick
frying pan to just cover the base. Add
the rounds in a single layer and cook
over moderate heat, about 4 minutes
each side or until browned.

MAKES 8 FRITTERS

Hot Potato Salad

*This tasty potato salad could be served
alongside grilled or barbecued meat.*

■

GLYCEMIC INDEX: 62
NUTRIENTS PER SERVING:

CALORIES 120
FAT . . . . .3 g
CARBOHYDRATE . . . . 16 g
FIBER . . . . .3 g

1. Boil unpeeled potatoes until just tender.

2. While the potatoes are cooking, cut the pepper, onion and zucchini into very fine slivers.

3. Mix mayonnaise, sour cream, mustard, garlic and lemon juice together.

4. Drain the potatoes and toss the hot, cooked potatoes in the dressing.

4. Make a bed of the raw vegetables on the serving plates and top with the hot potato salad.

SERVES 4

12 ozs. (about 12) tiny new potatoes, halved

½ (3 ozs.) pepper (any color)

½ red Spanish onion or 1 large shallot or scallion

1 small (4 ozs.) zucchini

1 tablespoon mayonnaise

1 tablespoon light sour cream

2 teaspoons grainy mustard

1 clove garlic, crushed

squeeze of lemon juice

Desserts

CRAN-APPLE CRISP

APPLE SHELL PUDDING

BAKED APPLES

CREAMED RICE WITH SLICED PEARS

CREAMY APRICOT SLICE

REFRESHING FRUIT CHEESECAKE

YOGURT BERRY JELL-O

WINTER FRUIT SALAD

APPLE CRUMBLE

■

Cran-Apple Crisp

*Apples, custard and a crispy topping make this
a popular year-round dessert.*

■

GLYCEMIC INDEX: 52
NUTRIENTS PER SERVING (SERVING 6):

CALORIES 287

FAT .... 9 g

CARBOHYDRATE .... 50 g

FIBER .... 4 g

1. Peel and core the apples and cut into thin slices. Drizzle with lemon juice. Microwave (100% power) for 5 to 8 minutes, or lightly stew in a saucepan, until just tender.

2. Add the cranberries. Place into a well-greased ovenproof dish.

3. Cook the pudding according to package directions. Pour over the apple mixture.

4. Melt the butter and honey in a small saucepan or in the microwave. Combine with the rolled oats, flour, spices and nuts. Sprinkle over the apple and pudding mixture.

5. Bake in a moderate oven (375°) for about 30 minutes or until the topping is browned.

SERVES 4 TO 6

4 medium to large Granny Smith apples (about 1 lb.)

juice of 1 lemon

1 cup cranberries, fresh or frozen

1 oz. package vanilla pudding mix

16 ozs. 1% milk

3 tablespoons butter

1½ tablespoons honey

1 cup (3 ozs.) rolled oats

¼ cup flour, sifted

1 teaspoon ground cinnamon

½ teaspoon ground allspice

1 tablespoon chopped walnuts or pecans

Apple Shell Pudding

*A different way to eat pasta and a good way to use up
leftover cooked pasta. Serve this accompanied
with a fresh fruit salad.*

■

GLYCEMIC INDEX: 41
NUTRIENTS PER SERVING:
CALORIES 220
FAT . . . . 4 g
CARBOHYDRATE . . . . 39 g
FIBER . . . . 2 g

2 *eggs*

3 *cups (1 lb.) cooked small
pasta shells*

½ *cup (3½ ozs.) sugar*

1 *teaspoon ground cinnamon*

½ *teaspoon allspice*

1 *cup (10 ozs.) grated apple*

1 *tablespoon butter, melted*

1. Whisk the eggs in a bowl until thick, add all the remaining ingredients. Stir until well combined.

2. Pour the mixture into a greased shallow baking dish. Bake in a moderate oven (350°) for about 40 minutes or until set in the center.

SERVES 6

*You will need to cook 1½ cups (9 ozs.)
pasta for this recipe.*

Baked Apples

Tender cooked apples, stuffed with plump dried fruits makes an easy low G.I. dessert.

■

GLYCEMIC INDEX: 45
NUTRIENTS PER SERVING:

CALORIES 246

FAT .... 4 g

CARBOHYDRATE .... 52 g

FIBER .... 4 g

1. Core the apples, keeping them whole. Remove the peel from around one end and in strips around each apple (to give a striped appearance).

2. Combine the currants, raisins, prunes, apricots, lemon zest, cinnamon and jam in a small bowl. Stuff the mixture into the apple centers.

3. Place the apples in a baking dish just large enough to hold them.

4. Combine the butter, honey, orange juice and nutmeg in a small saucepan. Stir over low heat until the butter is melted. Pour over the apples. Bake in a moderate oven (350°), for about 40 minutes, or until the apples are tender but not mushy, basting with the juices every 10 minutes.

5. Serve the apples drizzled with some of the juices from the dish.

SERVES 4

4 large golden delicious apples (1½ lbs.)

2 tablespoons raisins

4 prunes, pitted and chopped

4 dried apricots, chopped

½ teaspoon grated lemon zest

½ teaspoon ground cinnamon

1 tablespoon apricot jam

1½ tablespoons butter

¼ cup (2 ozs.) honey

6 tablespoons (3 ozs.) orange juice

½ teaspoon grated nutmeg

Creamed Rice with Sliced Pears

A yummy variation on creamed rice with an intermediate G.I.

■

GLYCEMIC INDEX: 56
NUTRIENTS PER SERVING:

CALORIES 290
FAT....................negligble
CARBOHYDRATE ....65 g
FIBER ....3 g

2 cups (16 ozs.) water

1 cup (6½ ozs.) long grain
rice

¾ cup (6 ozs.) evaporated
skim milk

¼ cup (2 ozs.) firmly packed
brown sugar

1 teaspoon vanilla extract

16 pear slices, canned or
fresh

1. Bring the water to a boil in a saucepan,
   add the rice and boil for 15 minutes;
   drain.

2. Return the rice to the saucepan with
   the milk. Stir over low heat until all
   the milk is absorbed. Stir in the sugar
   and vanilla extract; cool.

3. Using an ice cream scoop, serve scoops
   of rice with the pear slices.

SERVES 4

Creamy Apricot Slice

To toast coconut, cook in a nonstick frypan over low heat, stirring for 2 minutes or until just golden. Remove from the pan to cool.

▪

GLYCEMIC INDEX: 46
NUTRIENTS PER SERVING:

CALORIES 255

FAT . . . . 10 g

CARBOHYDRATE . . . . 38 g

FIBER . . . . 2 g

1. Line an 11 inch x 7 inch rectangular pan with foil.

2. For the base, combine the ingredients in a bowl and mix well. Press the mixture evenly over the base of the prepared pan.

3. Bake in a moderate oven (350°) for about 10 minutes or until browned. Remove from oven and allow to cool.

4. For the topping, cover the apricots with the boiling water, let stand 30 minutes or until soft. Process in a blender or food processor until smooth. Add the yogurt, honey and eggs and blend until smooth.

5. Spread the topping mixture over the prepared base. Bake in a moderate oven (350°) for about 30 to 35 minutes or until set.

6. Cool, then refrigerate several hours before serving.

SERVES 8

BASE

¼ cup (⅔ ozs.) desiccated coconut, toasted

5 ozs. graham cracker crumbs, finely crushed

4 tablespoons (2 ozs.) butter, melted

TOPPING

1 cup (4 ozs.) dried apricots

½ cup (4 ozs.) boiling water

2 6-oz. containers low fat apricot yogurt

¼ cup (2 ozs.) honey

2 eggs

Refreshing Fruit Cheesecake

A delicious lower fat cheesecake that leaves you feeling good after you eat it—not weighed down with fat.

■

GLYCEMIC INDEX: 53
NUTRIENTS PER SERVING:

CALORIES 304
FAT . . . . 13 g
CARBOHYDRATE . . . . 40 g
FIBER . . . . 1 g

BASE

8 ozs. graham cracker crumbs

6 tablespoons (3 ozs.) butter, melted

FILLING

2 teaspoons gelatin

2 tablespoons boiling water

6 ozs. low fat fruit yogurt

8 oz. carton low fat pineapple cottage cheese

¼ cup (2 ozs.) honey

½ teaspoon vanilla extract

1 cup (6½ ozs.) chopped fresh fruit (e.g. apple, orange, canteloupe, strawberries, pear, grapes)

1. For the base, combine the graham cracker crumbs and butter in a bowl. Press evenly into a 9 inch pie dish. Bake in a moderate oven (375°) for 10 minutes. Cool.

2. For the filling, sprinkle the gelatin over the boiling water in a cup, stand cup in a small pan of simmering water and stir until dissolved; cool slightly.

3. Process the cooled gelatin with the yogurt, cottage cheese, honey and vanilla extract in a blender or food processor until smooth.

4. Arrange the chopped fruit over the prepared crust and pour over the yogurt mixture. Refrigerate for about 1 hour or until set.

SERVES 8

Don't use papaya, pineapple or kiwi as these tend to prevent gelatin from setting.

Yogurt Berry Jell-O

An easy dessert. You could make it with sugar free Jell-O
if you wanted to reduce the calorie content.

■

GLYCEMIC INDEX: 54
NUTRIENTS PER SERVING:

CALORIES 111
FAT ....negligible
CARBOHYDRATE ....20 g
FIBER ....1 g

1. Combine the Jell-O and the boiling water in a bowl, stir until dissolved; cool but do not allow to set.

2. Coarsely chop the strawberries (frozen raspberries will tend to break up on stirring).

3. Fold the yogurt and berries through the Jell-O; mix well. Pour into serving cups and refrigerate until set.

SERVES 4

3 oz. package
berry-flavored Jell-O

1 cup (8 ozs.) boiling water

1 cup (5 ozs.) strawberries
or frozen raspberries

1½ cups (2 6-oz. containers)
low fat berry yogurt

Winter Fruit Salad
·

GLYCEMIC INDEX: 47
NUTRIENTS PER SERVING:

CALORIES 139
FAT ....1 g
CARBOHYDRATE ....33 g
FIBER ....5 g

1 orange, peeled and separated into segments

1 medium red apple, cut into bite-size cubes

2 teaspoons sugar

1 teaspoon fresh lemon juice

1 small banana

1 tablespoon shredded coconut

1. Cut orange segments in half. Place apple and orange chunks in a bowl. Sprinkle over the sugar and lemon juice and mix thoroughly. Cover and refrigerate at least 1 hour.

2. Just before serving, stir in the sliced banana. Sprinkle with coconut to serve.

SERVES 2

Apple Crumble

*A quick and easy version that makes
a delicious low G.I. dessert.*

■

GLYCEMIC INDEX: 51
NUTRIENTS PER SERVING:

CALORIES 360

FAT .... 12 g

CARBOHYDRATE .... 60 g

FIBER .... 7 g

1. Combine the apples and allspice and place in a 9 inch pie dish.

2. In a food processor combine the rest of the ingredients until crumbly.

3. Sprinkle over the apples. Bake in a 375° oven for 30 minutes.

SERVES 4 (GENEROUSLY)

*3 large Granny Smith
apples, peeled, cored and
sliced*

½ teaspoon allspice

CRUMBLE

1 cup (3 ozs.) rolled oats

*1¼ ozs. unprocessed oat
bran*

½ cup brown sugar

1 teaspoon cinnamon

*3 tablespoons (1½ ozs.)
butter*

Snacks

PITA PIZZETTE

CHICK NUTS

PEACH SMOOTHIE

CHEESE AND HERB OAT SCONES

SPICY BEAN DIP

LOW FAT GRANOLA BARS

MUESLI MUNCHIES

OAT AND APPLE MUFFINS

■

Pita Pizzette

A "good" snack must be quick and easy to make, taste great and not cause cravings. Here's a good snack—enjoy!

■

GLYCEMIC INDEX: 54
NUTRIENTS PER SERVING:
CALORIES 106
FAT . . . . .2 g
CARBOHYDRATE . . . . .17 g
FIBER . . . . .1 g

1. Place pita breads topside up on baking dish. Broil for 1 minute. Remove breads from oven and turn them over.

2. Equally divide remaining ingredients and arrange on the untoasted bottom sides of the pitas.

3. Place under broiler for 1 minute or until cheese melts. Serve immediately.

SERVES 4

4 1-oz. round mini pita breads

8 tablespoons tomato sauce

½ teaspoon dried oregano

8 tablespoons part skim mozzarella, shredded

Chick Nuts

A tasty low fat, low G.I. nibble. Spice them up with the suggested flavorings or experiment with your own combinations. All you need is some chickpeas.

■

GLYCEMIC INDEX: 33
1/2 CUP CHICKPEAS PROVIDING:

CALORIES 323
FAT .... 6 g
CARBOHYDRATE .... 45 g
FIBER .... 15 g

1 lb. package dried chick-peas

1. Soak the chickpeas in water overnight. Next day, drain and pat dry with paper towels.

2. Spread the chickpeas in a single layer baking pan. Bake in a moderate oven (375°) for about 45 minutes or until completely crisp. (They will shrink to their original size.)

3. Toss with a flavoring (see below) while hot, or cool and serve plain.

FLAVOR VARIATIONS

Chick Devils
Sprinkle a mixture of cayenne pepper and salt over the hot chick nuts.

Red Chicks
Sprinkle a mixture of paprika and garlic salt over the hot chick nuts.

MAKES 6 CUPS

After seasoning these, allow them to air dry for a few days to ensure all residual moisture has evaporated.

Peach Smoothie

Two straws in a tall frosted glass of this fruit beverage—
a low G.I. answer to a soda fountain soda!

■

GLYCEMIC INDEX: 19
NUTRIENTS PER SERVING:
CALORIES........................69
FAT........................0 g
CARBOHYDRATE.........,..14 g
FIBER......................1 g

1. Slice peach or drain canned peach slices.

2. In food processor, blend fruit and yogurt at high speed for 45 seconds.

3. Pour into 2 tall glasses. Serve immediately.

Note: Crushed ice and a sprinkle of cinnamon may be added if desired.

SERVES 2

1 medium peach, peeled, or ½ cup canned peaches, unsweetened

8 ozs. nonfat peach yogurt with artificial sweetener

ground cinnamon

Cheese and Herb Oat Scones

These savory scones make a delicious light lunch with salad or a tasty snack on their own. They are ready to eat as they are!

■

GLYCEMIC INDEX: 60
NUTRIENTS PER SCONE:
CALORIES 106
FAT .... 4 g
CARBOHYDRATE .... 19 g
FIBER .... 3 g

---

1 cup (5 ozs.) self-rising flour, sifted

1½ teaspoons baking powder

1 cup (4½ ozs.) unprocessed oat bran

2 tablespoons (1 oz.) butter

½ cup (4 ozs.) 2% milk

2 tablespoons water

½ cup (2 ozs.) grated low fat cheddar cheese

2 teaspoons chopped fresh parsley

2 teaspoons chopped fresh basil or 1 teaspoon dried basil leaves

1 teaspoon dried rosemary leaves

1. Sift the flour and baking powder into a large bowl, stir in the oat bran. Rub in the butter.

2. Make a well in the center and add the milk and half the water. Mix lightly with a knife, adding extra water if necessary, to make a soft dough. Turn the dough onto a lightly floured board and knead gently.

3. Roll out the dough into a rectangle about ⅓ inch thick. Scatter half the cheese and all the herbs over the entire surface.

4. Beginning from a long side, roll up to make a thick sausage. Cut into 1 inch slices to make little rounds.

5. Place the rounds side by side on a greased baking pan and sprinkle with the remaining cheese. Bake in a hot oven (400°) for about 20 minutes or until golden brown. Serve hot or cold.

MAKES 10 SCONES

Spicy Bean Dip

This dip is hot to taste but that's the appeal of it!
Use as a dip with crackers or as a tasty pasta sauce.

■

GLYCEMIC INDEX: 57
NUTRIENTS PER SERVING:

CALORIES 190
FAT ....3 g
CARBOHYDRATE ....25 g
FIBER ....7 g

1. Heat the oil in a nonstick frying pan or small saucepan. Add the onion and pepper and cook for about 5 minutes or until soft. Add the curry powder and chili and cook for 30 seconds.

2. Stir in the Worcestershire sauce, beans, tomato puree and wine. Bring to a boil.

3. Reduce heat and simmer, uncovered, for about 20 minutes or until thickened.

SERVES 4 AS A SAUCE

2 teaspoons olive oil

1 medium onion (4 ozs.), finely chopped

1 medium green pepper (5 ozs.), finely chopped

1 teaspoon curry powder

1 teaspoon minced jalapeno

2–3 teaspoons Worcestershire sauce

15½ oz. can kidney beans, drained

1 cup (8 ozs.) tomato puree

1 cup (8 ozs.) red wine

Low Fat Granola Bars

These bars have a heavy, wholesome texture and make a very sustaining snack if you are hungry.

■

GLYCEMIC INDEX: 54
NUTRIENTS PER BAR:

CALORIES 167
FAT . . . . .8 g
CARBOHYDRATE . . . . .15 g
FIBER . . . . .3 g

½ cup (2 ozs.) whole wheat flour

½ cup (2½ ozs.) self-rising flour

1 teaspoon baking powder

½ teaspoon allspice

½ teaspoon ground cinnamon

1½ cups (4 ozs.) rolled oats

1 cup (5 ozs.) dried fruit medley or dried fruit of choice, chopped

¼ cup (1 oz.) sunflower seed kernels

½ cup (4 ozs.) apple juice

¼ cup (2 ozs.) oil

1 egg, lightly beaten

2 egg whites, lightly beaten

1. Line an 8 x 12 inch pan with baking paper.

2. Sift the flours, baking powder and spices into a large bowl. Stir in the oats, fruit and seeds and stir to combine.

3. Add the apple juice, oil and whole egg; mix well. Gently mix in the egg whites until combined.

4. Press the mixture evenly into the prepared pan and press firmly with the back of a spoon. Mark the surface into 12 bars using a sharp knife.

5. Bake in a hot oven (400°) for about 15 to 20 minutes or until lightly browned. Cool and cut into bars.

MAKES 12 BARS

Muesli Munchies

*Crunchy little bite-sized biscuits which make
handy low G.I. snacks.*

■

GLYCEMIC INDEX: 56
NUTRIENTS PER BISCUIT:

CALORIES 134

FAT .... 7 g

CARBOHYDRATE .... 19 g

FIBER .... 2 g

1. Melt the butter and honey in a small saucepan.

2. Whisk the egg and vanilla extract together in a large bowl.

3. Add the butter mixture, muesli, sunflower seed kernels and flour to the egg mixture; stir until combined.

4. Place small spoonfuls of the mixture onto a lightly greased baking pan, spacing evenly.

5. Bake in a moderately hot oven (375°) for about 10 minutes or until golden brown. Let stand on pan until firm, then loosen and place on a wire rack to cool.

MAKES 16 COOKIES

*6 tablespoons (3 ozs.)
   butter*

¼ cup (2 ozs.) honey

1 egg

½ teaspoon vanilla extract

*2½ cups (10 ozs.) natural
   muesli*

*2 tablespoons sunflower
   seed kernels*

*¼ cup (1⅓ ozs.) self-rising
   flour, sifted*

Oat and Apple Muffins

These are a delicious low fat muffin, with moist chunks of apple through them.

■

GLYCEMIC INDEX: 56
NUTRIENTS PER MUFFIN:

CALORIES.........................93
FAT..........................1 g
CARBOHYDRATE............22 g
FIBER......................2 g

½ cup All-Bran cereal

⅔ cup (5½ ozs.) 1% milk

½ cup (2½ ozs.) self-rising flour

2 teaspoons baking powder

1 teaspoon allspice

½ cup (2½ ozs.) unprocessed oat bran

½ cup (2½ ozs.) raisins

1 green apple, peeled and diced

1 egg, lightly beaten

¼ cup (2 ozs.) honey

½ teaspoon vanilla extract

1. Combine the All-Bran and milk in a bowl and let stand for 10 minutes.

2. Sift the flour, baking powder and mixed spice into a large bowl. Stir in the oat bran, raisins and apple.

3. Combine the egg, honey and vanilla extract in a bowl. Add the egg mixture and All-Bran mixture to the dry ingredients and stir with a wooden spoon until just combined. Do not over mix.

4. Spoon the mixture into a greased 12-hole muffin tray. Bake in a moderate oven (375°) for about 15 minutes or until lightly browned and cooked through. Serve warm or at room temperature.

MAKES 12 MUFFINS

If you find them too dry when at room temperature, warm in the microwave (100% power) for 10 seconds before serving.

Warm the honey first to make measuring easy.

Part 3

THE GLYCEMIC INDEX TABLE

HOW TO USE THE GLYCEMIC INDEX TABLE

THE GLYCEMIC INDEX TABLE

■

HOW TO USE THE
GLYCEMIC INDEX TABLE

The following table is an A to Z listing of the glycemic index of commonly eaten foods in the United States and Canada. Approximately 300 different foods are listed. They include some new values for foods tested only recently.

The G.I. value shown next to each food is the average for that food using glucose as the standard, i.e., glucose has a G.I. value of 100, with other foods rated accordingly. The average may represent the mean of 10 studies of that food worldwide or only 2 to 4 studies. In a few instances, American data are different from the rest of the world and we show that data rather than the average. Rice and oatmeal fall into this category.

To check on a food's glycemic index, simply look for it by name in the alphabetic list. You may also find it under a food type—fruit, cookies.

Included in the tables is the carbohydrate (CHO) and fat content of a *sample* serving of the food. This is to help you keep track of the amount of fat and carbohydrate in your diet. The sample serving is not the recommended serving—it is just an example of a serving. The glycemic index does not depend on your serving size because it is a ranking of the glycemic effect of foods using carbohydrate-equivalent portion sizes. You can eat **more** of a low G.I. food or **less** of a high G.I. food and achieve the same blood sugar levels.

Remember when you are choosing foods, the glycemic index isn't the only thing to consider. In terms of your blood sugar levels you should also consider the amount of carbohydrate you are eating. For your overall health the fat, fiber and micronutrient content of your diet is also important. A dietitian can guide you further with good food choices; see page 15 for advice on finding a dietitian.

FOR A SMALL EATER, AIM FOR LESS THAN 50 G FAT A DAY

AND MORE THAN 200 G CARBOHYDRATE.

FOR A BIGGER EATER, AIM FOR LESS THAN 80 G FAT A DAY

AND MORE THAN 300 G CARBOHYDRATE.

A–Z OF FOODS
WITH GLYCEMIC INDEX, CARBOHYDRATE & FAT

Food	Glycemic Index	Fat (g per serving)	CHO (g per serving)
Agave nectar (90% fructose syrup), 1 tablespoon	11	0	16
All-Bran with extra fiber™, Kellogg's, breakfast cereal, ½ cup, 1 oz.	51 (av)	1	22
Angel food cake, ¹⁄₁₂ cake, 1 oz.	67	trace	17
Apple, 1 medium, 5 ozs.	38 (av)	0	18
Apple, dried, 1 oz.	29	0	24
Apple juice, unsweetened, 1 cup, 8 ozs.	40	0	29
Apple cinnamon muffin, from mix, 1 muffin,	44	5	26
Apricots, fresh, 3 medium, 3 ozs.	57	0	12
canned, light syrup, 3 halves	64	0	14
dried, 5 halves	31	0	13
Apricot Jam, no added sugar, 1 tablespoon	55	0	17
Apricot and honey muffin, low fat, from mix, 1 muffin	60	4	27
Bagel, 1 small, plain, 2.3 ozs.	72	1	38
Baked beans, ½ cup, 4 ozs.	48 (av)	1	24
Banana bread, 1 slice, 3 ozs.	47	7	46
Banana, raw, 1 medium, 5 ozs.	55 (av)	0	32
Banana, oat and honey muffin, low fat from mix, 1 muffin	65	4	27
Barley, pearled, boiled, ½ cup, 2.6 ozs.	25 (av)	0	22
Basmati white rice, boiled, 1 cup, 6 ozs.	58	0	50
Beets, canned, drained, ½ cup, 3 ozs.	64	0	5
Black bean soup, ½ cup, 4.5 ozs.	64	2	19
Black beans, boiled, ¾ cup, 4.3 ozs.	30	1	31
Black bread, dark rye, 1 slice, 1.7 ozs.	76	1	18
Blackeyed peas, canned, ½ cup, 4 ozs.	42	1	16
Blueberry muffin, 1 muffin, 2 ozs.	59	4	27
Bran			
All-Bran with extra fiber™, Kellogg's, ½ cup, 1 oz.	51	1	20
Bran Buds with Psyllium™, Kellogg's, ⅓ cup, 1 oz.	45	1	24
Bran Flakes, Post, ⅔ cup, 1 oz.	74	1	22

Food	Glycemic Index	Fat (g per serving)	CHO (g per serving)
Oat bran, 1 tablespoon	55	1	7
Oat bran muffin, 2 ozs.	60	4	28
Rice bran, 1 tablespoon	19	2	5
Breads			
Dark rye, Black bread, 1 slice, 1.7 ozs.	76	1	18
Dark rye, Schinkenbröt, 1 slice, 2 ozs.	86	1	22
Eagle Mills Bread Mix—Muesli with Sustagrain™, 2 ozs.	54	1	24
Eagle Mills Bread Mix—Soy with Flaxseed™, 2 ozs.	50	1	17
French baguette, 1 oz.	95	1	15
Gluten-free bread, 1 slice, 1 oz.	90	1	18
Hamburger bun, 1 prepacked bun, 1.5 ozs.	61	2	22
Kaiser roll, 1, 2 ozs.	73	2	34
Light deli (American) rye, 1 slice, 1 oz.	68	1	16
Melba toast, 6 pieces, 1 oz.	70	2	23
Pita bread, whole wheat, 6 ½ inch loaf, 2 ozs.	57	2	35
Pumpernickel, whole grain, 1 slice, 1 oz.	51	1	15
Rye bread, 1 slice, 1 oz.	65	1	15
Sourdough, 1 slice, 1.5 ozs.	52	1	20
Sourdough rye, Arnold's, 1 slice, 1.5 ozs.	57	1	21
White, 1 slice, 1 oz.	70 (av)	1	12
100% stoneground whole wheat, 1 slice, 1.5 ozs.	53	1	15
Whole wheat, 1 slice, 1 oz.	69 (av)	1	13
Bread stuffing from mix, 2 ozs.	74	5	13
Breakfast cereals			
All-Bran with extra fiber™, Kellogg's, ½ cup, 1 oz.	51	1	20
Bran Buds with Psyllium™, Kellogg's, ⅓ cup, 1 oz.	45	1	24
Bran Flakes, Post, ⅔ cup, 1 oz.	74	1	22
Cheerios ™, General Mills, 1 cup, 1 oz.	74	2	23
Cocoa Krispies™, Kellogg's, 1 cup, 1 oz.	77	1	27
Corn Bran™, Quaker Crunchy, ¾ cup, 1 oz.	75	1	23
Corn Chex™, Nabisco, 1 cup, 1 oz.	83	0	26
Corn Flakes™, Kellogg's, 1 cup, 1 oz.	84 (av)	0	24
Crispix™, Kellogg's, 1 cup, 1 oz.	87	0	25

Food	Glycemic Index	Fat (g per serving)	CHO (g per serving)
Frosted Flakes™, Kellogg's, ¾ cup, 1 oz.	55	0	28
Grapenuts™, Post, ¼ cup, 1 oz.	67	1	27
Grapenuts Flakes™, Post, ¾ cup, 1 oz.	80	1	24
Life™, Quaker, ¾ cup, 1 oz.	66	1	25
Muesli, natural muesli, ⅔ cup, 1.5 ozs.	56	3	28
Muesli, toasted, ⅔ cup, 2 ozs.	43	10	41
Oat bran, raw, 1 tablespoon	55	1	7
Oat bran™, Quaker Oats, breakfast cereal, ¾ cup, 1 oz.	50	1	23
Oatmeal (made with water), old fashioned, cooked, ½ cup, 4 ozs.	49 (av)	1	12
Puffed Wheat™, Quaker, 2 cups, 1 oz.	67	0	22
Raisin Bran™, Kellogg's, ¾ cup, 1 oz.	73	0	32
Rice bran, 1 tablespoon	19	2	5
Rice Chex™, General Mills, 1¼ cups, 1 oz.	89	0	27
Rice Krispies™, Kellogg's, 1¼ cups, 1 oz.	82	0	26
Shredded wheat, spoonsize, ⅔ cup, 1.2 oz.	58	0	27
Shredded Wheat™, Post, 1 oz.	67	1	23
Smacks™, Kellogg's, ¾ cup, 1 oz.	56	1	24
Special K™, Kellogg's, 1 cup, 1 oz.	54	0	22
Team Flakes™, Nabisco, ¾ cup, 1 oz.	82	0	25
Total™, General Mills, ¾ cup, 1 oz.	76	1	24
WeetaBix™, 2 biscuits, 1.2 ozs.	75	1	28
Buckwheat groats, cooked, ½ cup, 2.7 ozs.	54 (av)	1	20
Bulgur, cooked, ⅔ cup, 4 ozs.	48 (av)	0	23
Bun, hamburger, 1 prepacked bun, 1.7 ozs.	61	2	22
Butter beans, boiled, ½ cup, 4 ozs.	31 (av)	0	16
Cakes			
Angel food cake, 1 slice, 1/12 cake, 1 oz.	67	trace	17
Banana bread, 1 slice, 3 ozs.	47	7	46
Pound cake, homemade, 1 slice, 3 ozs.	54	15	42
Sponge cake, 1 slice, 1/12 cake, 2 ozs.	46	4	32
Capellini pasta, cooked, 1 cup, 6 ozs.	45	1	53
Canteloupe, raw, ¼ small, 6.5 ozs.	65	0	16

Food	Glycemic Index	Fat (g per serving)	CHO (g per serving)
Carrots, peeled, boiled, canned, ½ cup, 2.4 ozs.	49	0	3
Cereal grains			
Barley, pearled, boiled, ½ cup, 2.6 ozs.	25 (av)	0	22
Bulgur, cooked, ½ cup, 3 ozs.	48 (av)	0	17
Couscous, cooked, ½ cup, 3 ozs.	65 (av)	0	21
Corn			
Cornmeal, whole grain, from mix, cooked,			
⅓ cup, 1.4 ozs.	68	1	30
Sweet corn, canned, drained, ½ cup, 3 ozs.	55 (av)	1	15
Taco shells, 2 shells, 1 oz.	68	5	17
Rice			
Basmati, white, boiled, 1 cup, 6 ozs.	58	0	50
Brown, 1 cup, 6 ozs.	55 (av)	0	37
Converted™, Uncle Ben's, 1 cup, 6 ozs.	44	0	38
Instant, cooked, 1 cup, 6 ozs.	87	0	37
Long grain, white, 1 cup, 6 ozs.	56 (av)	0	42
Parboiled, 1 cup, 6ozs.	48	0	38
Rice bran, 1 tablespoon	19	2	5
Rice cakes, plain, 3 cakes, 1 oz.	82	1	23
Short grain, white, 1 cup, 6 ozs.	72	0	42
Chana dal, ½ cup, 4 ozs.	8	3	28
Cheerios™, General Mills, breakfast cereal, 1 cup, 1 oz.	74	2	23
Cherries, 10 large cherries, 3 ozs.	22	0	10
Chickpeas (garbanzo beans),			
canned, drained, ½ cup, 4 ozs.	42	2	15
boiled, ½ cup, 3 ozs.	33 (av)	2	23
Chocolate butterscotch muffin, low fat from mix,			
1 muffin	53	4	29
Chocolate, bar, 1.5 ozs.	49	14	26
Chocolate Nestle Quik™ (made with water),			
3 teaspoons	53	0	14
Coca-Cola™, soft drink, 1 can	63	0	39
Cocoa Krispies™, Kellogg's, breakfast cereal, 1 cup,			
1 oz.	77	1	27

Food	Glycemic Index	Fat (g per serving)	CHO (g per serving)
Corn			
Cornmeal, cooked from mix, ⅓ cup, 1.4 ozs.	68	1	30
Sweet corn, canned and drained, ½ cup, 3 ozs.	55 (av)	1	15
Corn Bran™, Quaker Crunchy, breakfast cereal, ¾ cup, 1 oz.	75	1	23
Corn Chex™, General Mills, breakfast cereal, 1 cup, 1 oz.	83	0	26
Corn chips, 1 oz.	72	10	16
Corn Flakes, Kellogg's, breakfast cereal, 1 cup, 1 oz.	84 (av)	0	24
Cornmeal, from mix, cooked, ⅓ cup, 1.4 ozs.	68	1	30
Cookies			
Graham crackers, 4 squares, 1 oz.	74	3	22
Milk Arrowroot, 3 cookies, ½ oz.	69	2	9
Oatmeal, 1 cookie, ⅔ oz.	55	3	12
Shortbread, 4 small cookies, 1 oz.	64	7	19
Social Tea™ biscuits, Nabisco, 4 cookies, ⅔ oz.	55	3	13
Vanilla wafers, 7 cookies, 1 oz.	77	4	21
see also Crackers			
Couscous, cooked, ⅔ cup, 4 ozs.	65 (av)	0	21
Crackers			
Crispbread, 3 crackers, ⅔ oz.	81	0	15
Kavli™ whole grain crispbread, 4 wafers, 1 oz.	71	1	16
Premium soda crackers, saltine, 8 crackers, 1 oz.	74	3	17
Rice cakes, plain, 3 cakes, 1 oz.	82	1	23
Ryvita™ tasty dark rye whole grain crispbread, 2 slices, ⅔ oz.	69	1	16
Stoned wheat thins, 3 crackers, ⅘ oz.	67	2	15
Water cracker, Carr's, 3 king size crackers, ⅘ oz.	78	2	18
Crispix™, Kellogg's, breakfast cereal, 1 cup, 1 oz.	87	0	25
Croissant, medium, 1.2 ozs.	67	14	27
Dairy foods and nondairy substitutes			
Ice cream, 10% fat, vanilla, ½ cup, 2.2 ozs.	61 (av)	7	16

Food	Glycemic Index	Fat (g per serving)	CHO (g per serving)
Ice milk, vanilla, ½ cup, 2.2 ozs.	50	3	15
Milk, whole, 1 cup, 8 ozs.	27 (av)	9	11
skim, 1 cup, 8 ozs.	32	0	12
chocolate flavored, 1%, 1 cup, 8 ozs.	34	3	26
Pudding, ½ cup, 4.4 ozs.	43	4	24
Soy milk, 1 cup, 8 ozs.	31	7	14
Tofu frozen dessert (nondairy), low fat, ½ cup, 2 ozs.	115	1	21
Yogurt			
nonfat, fruit flavored, with sugar, 8 ozs.	33	0	30
nonfat, plain, artificial sweetener, 8 ozs.	14	0	17
nonfat, fruit flavored, artificial sweetener, 8 ozs.	14	0	16
Dates, dried, 5, 1.4 ozs.	103	0	27
Doughnut with cinnamon and sugar, 1.6 ozs.	76	11	29
Fanta™, soft drink, 1 can	68	0	47
Fava beans, frozen, boiled, ½ cup, 3 ozs.	79	0	17
Fettucini, cooked, 1 cup, 6 ozs.	32	1	57
Fish sticks, frozen, oven-cooked, fingers, 3.5 ozs.	38	14	24
Flan cake, ½ cup, 4 ozs.	65	5	23
French baguette bread, 1 oz.	95	0	15
French fries, large, 4.3 ozs.	75	22	46
Frosted Flakes™, Kellogg's, breakfast cereal, ¾ cup, 1 oz.	55	0	28
Fructose, pure, 3 packets	23 (av)	0	10
Fruit cocktail, canned in natural juice, ½ cup, 4 ozs.	55	0	15
Fruits and fruit products			
Agave nectar (90% fructose syrup), 1 tablespoon	11	0	16
Apple, 1 medium, 5 ozs.	38 (av)	0	18
Apple, dried, 1 oz.	29	0	24
Apple juice, unsweetened, 1 cup, 8 ozs.	40	0	29
Apricots, fresh, 3 medium, 3.3 ozs.	57	0	12
canned, light syrup, 3 halves	64	0	19
dried, 1 oz.	31	0	13
Apricot jam, no added sugar, 1 tablespoon	55	0	17

Food	Glycemic Index	Fat (g per serving)	CHO (g per serving)
Banana, raw, 1 medium, 5 ozs.	55 (av)	0	32
Canteloupe, raw, ¼ small, 6.5 ozs.	65	0	16
Cherries, 10 large, 3 ozs.	22	0	10
Dates, dried, 5, 1.4 ozs.	103	0	27
Fruit cocktail, canned in natural juice, ½ cup, 4 ozs.	55	0	15
Grapefruit, raw, ½ medium, 3.3 ozs.	25	0	5
Grapefruit juice, unsweetened, 1 cup, 8 ozs.	48	0	22
Grapes, green, 1 cup, 3 ozs.	46 (av)	0	15
Kiwi, 1 medium, raw, peeled, 2.5 ozs.	52 (av)	0	8
Mango, 1 small, 5 ozs.	55 (av)	0	19
Marmalade, 1 tablespoon	48	0	17
Orange, navel, 1 medium, 4 ozs.	44 (av)	0	10
Orange juice, 1 cup, 8 ozs.	46	0	26
Papaya, ½ medium, 5 ozs.	58 (av)	0	14
Peach, fresh, 1 medium, 3 ozs.	42 (av)	0	7
canned, natural juice, ½ cup, 4 ozs.	30	0	14
canned, light syrup, ½ cup, 4 ozs.	52	0	18
canned, heavy syrup, ½ cup, 4 ozs.	58	0	26
Pear, fresh, 1 medium, 5 ozs.	38 (av)	0	21
canned in pear juice, ½ cup, 4 ozs.	44	0	13
Pineapple, fresh, 2 slices, 4 ozs.	66	0	10
Pineapple juice, unsweetened, canned, 8 ozs.	46	0	34
Plums, 1 medium, 2 ozs.	39 (av)	0	7
Raisins, ¼ cup, 1 oz.	64	0	28
Strawberry jam, 1 tablespoon	51	0	18
Watermelon, 1 cup, 5 ozs.	72	0	8
Gatorade™ sports drink, 1 cup, 8 ozs.	78	0	14
Glucose powder, 2½ tablets	102	0	10
Gluten-free bread, 1 slice, 1 oz.	90	1	18
Granola Bars™, Quaker Chewy, 1 oz.	61	2	23
Gnocchi, cooked, 1 cup, 5 ozs.	68	3	71
Graham crackers, 4 squares, 1 oz.	74	3	22
Grapefruit, raw, ½ medium, 3.3 ozs.	25	0	5
Grapefruit juice, unsweetened, 1 cup, 8 ozs.	48	0	22

Food	Glycemic Index	Fat (g per serving)	CHO (g per serving)
Grapenuts™, Post, breakfast cereal, ¼ cup, 1 oz.	67	1	27
Grapenuts Flakes™, Post, breakfast cereal, ¾ cup, 1 oz.	80	1	24
Grapes, green, 1 cup, 3.3 ozs.	46 (av)	0	15
Green pea soup, canned, ready to serve, 1 cup, 9 ozs.	66	3	27
Hamburger bun, 1 prepacked bun, 1.5 ozs.	61	2	22
Honey, 1 tablespoon	58	0	16
Ice cream, 10% fat, vanilla, ½ cup, 2.2 ozs.	61 (av)	7	16
Ice milk, vanilla, ½ cup, 2.2 ozs.	50	3	15
Isotar, 1 cup, 8 ozs.	73	0	18
Jelly beans, 10 large, 1 oz.	80	0	26
Kaiser rolls, 1 roll, 2 ozs.	73	2	34
Kavli™ whole grain crispbread, 4 wafers, 1 oz.	71	1	16
Kidney beans, red, boiled, ½ cup, 3 ozs.	27 (av)	0	20
Kidney beans, red, canned and drained, ½ cup, 4.3 ozs.	52	0	19
Kiwi, 1 medium, raw, peeled, 2.5 ozs.	52 (av)	0	8
Kudos Granola Bars™ (whole grain), 1 bar, 1 oz.	62	5	20
Lactose, pure, 1 oz.	46 (av)	0	10
Lentil soup, canned, 1 cup, 8 ozs.	44	1	24
Lentils, green and brown, boiled, ½ cup, 3 ozs.	30 (av)	0	16
Lentils, red, boiled, 1.4 cup, 4 ozs.	26 (av)	0	27
Life™, Quaker, breakfast cereal, ¾ cup, 1 oz.	66	1	25
Life Savers™, 6 pieces, peppermint	70	0	10
Light deli (American) rye bread, 1 slice, 1 oz.	68	1	16
Lima beans, baby, frozen, ½ cup, 3 ozs.	32	0	17
Linguine pasta, thick, cooked, 1 cup, 6 ozs.	46 (av)	1	56
Linguine pasta, thin, cooked, 1 cup, 6 ozs.	55 (av)	1	56
M & M's Chocolate Candies Peanut™, 1.7 oz. package	33	13	30
Macaroni and Cheese Dinner™, Kraft packaged, cooked, 1 cup, 7 ozs.	64	17	48
Macaroni, cooked, 1 cup, 6 ozs.	45	1	52
Maltose (maltodextrin), pure, 2½ teaspoons	105	0	10
Mango, 1 small, 5 ozs.	55 (av)	0	19

Food	Glycemic Index	Fat (g per serving)	CHO (g per serving)
Marmalade, 1 tablespoon	48	0	17
Mars Almond Bar™, 1.8 ozs.	65	12	31
Melba toast, 6 pieces, 1 oz.	70	2	23
Milk, whole, 1 cup, 8 ozs.	27 (av)	9	11
skim, 1 cup, 8 ozs.	32	0	12
chocolate flavored, 1%, 1 cup, 8 ozs.	34	3	26
Milk Arrowroot, 3 cookies, ½ oz.	63	2	9
Millet, cooked, ½ cup, 4 ozs.	71	1	28
Muesli, breakfast cereal toasted, ⅔ cup, 2 ozs.	43	10	41
non-toasted, ⅔ cup, 1.5 ozs.	56	3	28
Muffins			
Apple cinnamon, from mix, 1 muffin, 2 ozs.	44	8	33
Apricot and honey, low fat, from mix, 1 muffin	60	4	27
Banana, oat and honey, low fat, from mix, 1 muffin	65	4	27
Blueberry, 1 muffin, 2 ozs.	59	4	27
Chocolate butterscotch, low fat, from mix, 1 muffin	53	4	29
Oat and raisin, low fat, from mix, 1 muffin	54	3	28
Oat bran, 1 muffin, 2 ozs.	60	4	28
Mung beans, boiled, ½ cup, 3.5 ozs.	38	1	18
Navy beans, boiled, ½ cup, 3 ozs.	38 (av)	0	19
Nutella™ (spread), 2 tablespoons, 1 oz.	33	9	19
Oat and raisin muffin, low fat from mix, 1 muffin	54	3	28
Oat bran, 1 tablespoon	55	1	7
Oat bran™, Quaker Oats, breakfast cereal, ¾ cup, 1 oz.	50	1	23
Oat bran, 1 muffin, 2 ozs.	60	4	28
Oatmeal (made with water), old fashioned, cooked, 1 cup, 8 ozs.	49	2	26
Oatmeal cookie, 1, ⅖ oz.	55	3	12
Orange, navel, 1 medium, 4 ozs.	44 (av)	0	10
Orange syrup, diluted, 1 cup	66	0	20
Orange juice, 1 cup, 8 ozs.	46	0	26
Papaya, ½ medium, 5 ozs.	58 (av)	0	14
Parsnips, boiled, ½ cup, 2.5 ozs.	97	0	15

Food	Glycemic Index	Fat (g per serving)	CHO (g per serving)
Pasta			
Capellini, cooked, 1 cup, 6 ozs.	45	1	53
Fettucini, cooked, 1 cup, 6 ozs.	32	1	57
Gnocchi, cooked, 1 cup, 5 ozs.	68	3	71
Linguine thick, cooked, 1 cup, 6 ozs.	46 (av)	1	56
Linguine thin, cooked, 1 cup, 6 ozs.	55 (av)	1	56
Macaroni, cooked, 1 cup, 5 ozs.	45	1	52
Macaroni and Cheese Dinner™, Kraft, packaged, cooked, 1 cup, 7 ozs.	64	17	48
Ravioli, meat-filled, cooked, 1 cup, 9 ozs.	39	8	32
Rice vermicelli, cooked, 6 ozs.	58	0	48
Spaghetti, white, cooked, 1 cup, 6 ozs.	41 (av)	1	52
Spaghetti, whole wheat, cooked, 1 cup, 6 ozs.	37 (av)	1	48
Spirali, durum, cooked, 1 cup, 6 ozs.	43	1	56
Star Pastina, cooked, 1 cup, 6 ozs.	38	1	56
Tortellini, cheese, cooked, 8 ozs.	50	6	26
Vermicelli, cooked, 1 cup, 6 ozs.	35	0	42
Pastry, flaky, ⅛ of double crust, 2 ozs.	59	15	24
Pea soup, split with ham, canned, 1 cup, 5.5 ozs.	66	7	56
Peach, fresh, 1 medium, 3 ozs.	42 (av)	0	7
canned, heavy syrup, ½ cup, 4 ozs.	58	0	26
canned, light syrup, ½ cup, 4 ozs.	52	0	18
canned, natural juice, ½ cup, 4 ozs.	30	0	14
Peanuts, roasted, salted, ½ cup, 2.5 ozs.	14 (av)	38	16
Pear, fresh, 1 medium, 5 ozs.	38 (av)	0	21
canned in pear juice, ½ cup, 4 ozs.	44	0	13
Peas, green, fresh, frozen, boiled, ½ cup, 2.7 ozs.	48 (av)	0	11
Peas dried, boiled, ½ cup, 2 ozs.	22	0	7
Pineapple, fresh, 2 slices, 4 ozs.	66	0	10
Pineapple juice, unsweetened, canned, 8 ozs.	46	0	34
Pinto beans, canned, ½ cup, 4 ozs.	45	1	18
Pinto beans, soaked, boiled, ½ cup, 3 ozs.	39	0	22
Pita bread, whole wheat, 6 ½ inch loaf, 2 ozs.	57	2	35
Pizza, cheese and tomato, 2 slices, 8 ozs.	60	22	56

FOOD	GLYCEMIC INDEX	FAT (G PER SERVING)	CHO (G PER SERVING)
Plums, 1 medium, 2 ozs.	39 (av)	0	7
Popcorn, light, microwave, 2 cups (popped)	55	3	12
Potatoes			
Desirée, peeled, boiled, 1 medium, 4 ozs.	101	0	13
French fries, large, 4.3 ozs.	75	26	49
instant mashed potato, Carnation Foods™, ½ cup, 3.5 ozs.	86	2	14
new, unpeeled, boiled, 5 small (cocktail), 6 ozs.	62 (av)	0	23
new, canned, drained, 5 small, 6 ozs.	61	0	23
red-skinned, peeled, boiled, 1 medium, 4 ozs.	88 (av)	0	15
red-skinned, baked in oven (no fat), 1 medium, 4 ozs.	93 (av)	0	15
red-skinned, mashed, ½ cup, 4 ozs.	91 (av)	0	16
red-skinned, microwaved, 1 medium, 4 ozs.	79	0	15
sweet potato, peeled, boiled, ½ cup mashed, 3 ozs.	54 (av)	0	20
white-skinned, peeled, boiled, 1 medium, 4 ozs.	63 (av)	0	24
white-skinned, with skin, baked in oven (no fat), 1 medium, 4 ozs.	85 (av)	0	30
white-skinned, mashed, ½ cup, 4 ozs.	70 (av)	0	20
white-skinned, with skin, microwaved, 1 medium, 4 ozs.	82	0	29
Sebago, peeled, boiled, 1 medium, 4 ozs.	87	0	13
Potato chips, plain, 14 pieces, 1 oz.	54 (av)	11	15
Pound cake, 1 slice, homemade, 3 ozs.	54	15	42
Power Bar™, Performance, Chocolate, 1 bar	58	2	45
Premium saltine crackers, 8 crackers, 1 oz.	74	3	17
Pretzels, 1 oz.	83	1	22
Pudding, ½ cup, 4.4 ozs.	43	4	24
Puffed Wheat™, Quaker, breakfast cereal, 2 cups, 1 oz.	67	0	22
Pumpernickel bread, whole grain, 1 slice	51	1	15
Pumpkin, peeled, boiled, mashed, ½ cup, 4 ozs.	75	0	6
Raisins, ¼ cup, 1 oz.	64	0	28
Raisin Bran™, Kellogg's, breakfast cereal, ¾ cup, 1.3 ozs.	73	0	32

Food	Glycemic Index	Fat (g per serving)	CHO (g per serving)
Ravioli, meat-filled, cooked, 1 cup, 9 ozs.	39	8	32
Rice			
Basmati, white, boiled, 1 cup, 7 ozs.	58	0	50
Brown, 1 cup, 6 ozs.	55 (av)	0	37
Converted™, Uncle Ben's, 1 cup, 6 ozs.	44	0	38
Instant, cooked, 1 cup, 6 ozs.	87	0	37
Long grain, white, 1 cup, 6 ozs.	56 (av)	0	42
Parboiled, 1 cup, 6 ozs.	48	0	38
Rice bran, 1 tablespoon	19	2	5
Rice cakes, plain, 3 cakes, 1 oz.	82	1	23
Rice vermicelli, cooked, 6 ozs.	58	0	48
Short grain, white, 1 cup, 6 ozs.	72	0	42
Rice Chex™, General Mills, breakfast cereal, 1¼ cups, 1 oz.	89	0	27
Rice Krispies™, Kellogg's, breakfast cereal, 1¼ cups, 1 oz.	82	0	26
Rice vermicelli, cooked, 6 ozs.	58	0	48
Roll (bread), Kaiser, 1 roll, 2 ozs.	73	2	39
Romano (cranberry) beans, boiled, ½ cup, 3 ozs.	46	0	21
Rutabaga, peeled, boiled, ½ cup, 2.6 ozs.	72	0	3
Rye bread, 1 slice, 1 oz.	65	1	15
Ryvita™ tasty dark rye whole grain crispbread, 2 slices, ⅔ oz.	69	1	16
Sausages, smoked link, pork and beef, fried, 2.5 ozs.	28	29	5
Semolina, cooked, ⅔ cup, 6 ozs.	55	0	17
Shortbread, 4 small cookies, 1 oz.	64	7	19
Shredded Wheat™, Post, breakfast cereal, 1 oz.	83	1	23
Shredded wheat, 1 biscuit, ⅘ oz.	62	0	19
Skittles Original Fruit Bite Size Candies™, 2.3 oz. pk.	70	3	59
Smacks™, Kellogg's, breakfast cereal, ¾ cup, 1 oz.	56	1	24
Snickers™, 2.2 oz. bar	41	15	36
Social Tea™ Biscuits, Nabisco, 4 cookies, ⅔ oz.	55	3	13
Soft drink, Fanta™, 1 can, 12 ozs.	68	0	47

Food	Glycemic Index	Fat (g per serving)	CHO (g per serving)
Soups			
Black bean soup, ½ cup, 4.5 ozs.	64	2	19
Green pea soup, canned, ready to serve, 1 cup, 9 ozs.	66	3	27
Lentil soup, canned, 1 cup, 8 ozs.	44	1	24
Pea soup, split, with ham, 1 cup, 5.5 ozs.	66	7	56
Tomato soup, canned, 1 cup, 9 ozs.	38	4	33
Sourdough bread, 1 slice, 1.5 ozs.	52	1	20
rye bread, Arnold's, 1 slice, 1.5 ozs.	57	1	21
Soy beans, boiled, ½ cup, 3 ozs.	18 (av)	7	10
Soy milk, 1 cup, 8 ozs.	31	7	14
Spaghetti, white, cooked, 1 cup	41 (av)	1	52
Spaghetti, whole wheat, cooked, 1 cup, 5 ozs.	37 (av)	1	48
Special K™, Kellogg's, breakfast cereal, 1 cup, 1 oz.	54	0	22
Spirali, durum, cooked, 1 cup, 6 ozs.	43	1	56
Split pea soup, 8 ozs.	60	4	38
Split peas, yellow, boiled, ½ cup, 3.5 ozs.	32	0	21
Sponge cake plain, 1 slice, 3.5 ozs.	46	4	32
Sports drinks			
Gatorade™ 1 cup, 8 ozs.	78	0	14
Isostar, 1 cup, 8 ozs.	73	0	18
Sportsplus, 1 cup, 8 ozs.	74	0	17
Sports bars			
Power Bar™, Performance, chocolate, 1 bar	58	2	45
Stoned wheat thins, 3 crackers, ⅘ oz.	67	2	15
Strawberry Nestle Quik™ (made with water), 3 teaspoons	64	0	14
Strawberry jam, 1 tablespoon	51	0	18
Sucrose, 1 teaspoon	65 (av)	0	4
Syrup, fruit flavored, diluted, 1 cup	66	0	20
Sweet corn, canned, drained, ½ cup, 3 ozs.	55 (av)	1	16
Sweet potato, peeled, boiled, ½ cup mashed, 3 ozs.	54 (av)	0	20
Taco shells, 2 shells, 1 oz.	68	5	17

Food	Glycemic Index	Fat (g per serving)	CHO (g per serving)
Tapioca pudding, boiled with whole milk, 1 cup, 10 ozs.	81	13	51
Taro, peeled, boiled, ½ cup, 2 ozs.	54	0	23
Team Flakes™, Nabisco, breakfast cereal, ¾ cup, 1 oz.	82	0	25
Tofu frozen dessert, nondairy, low fat, 2 ozs.	115	1	21
Tomato soup, canned, 1 cup, 9 ozs.	38	4	33
Tortellini, cheese, cooked, 8 ozs.	50	6	26
Total™, General Mills, breakfast cereal, ¾ cup, 1 oz.	76	1	24
Twix Chocolate Caramel Cookie™, 2, 2 ozs.	44	14	37
Vanilla wafers, 7 cookies, 1 oz.	77	4	21
Vermicelli, cooked, 1 cup, 6 ozs.	35	0	42
Waffles, plain, frozen, 4 inch square, 1 oz.	76	3	13
Water crackers, 3 king size crackers, ⅘ oz.	78	2	18
Watermelon, 1 cup, 5 ozs.	72	0	8
Weetabix™ breakfast cereal, 2 biscuits, 1.2 ozs.	75	1	28
White bread, 1 slice, 1 oz.	70 (av)	1	12
Whole wheat bread, 1 slice, 1 oz.	69 (av)	1	13
Yam, boiled, 3 ozs.	51	0	31
Yogurt			
nonfat, fruit flavored, with sugar, 8 ozs.	33	0	30
nonfat, plain, artificial sweetener, 8 ozs.	14	0	17
nonfat, fruit flavored, artificial sweetener, 8 ozs.	14	0	16

GENERAL READING:

SOURCES AND REFERENCES

1 Jenkins DJA, Wolever TMS, Taylor RH, et al. *Glycemic index of foods: a physiological basis for carbohydrate exchange.* Am J Clin Nutr 1981; 34: 362–6.

2 Brand Miller J. (1994) *The importance of glycemic index in diabetes.* Am J Clin Nutr, 59 (suppl: 747S-752S).

3 Wolever TMS, Jenkins DJA, Jenkins AL, Josse RG. *The glycemic index: methodology and clinical implications.* Am J Clin Nutr 1991; 54: 846–54.

4 Jenkins DJA, Wolever TMS, Kalmusky J, et al. *Low glycemic index carbohydrate foods in the management of hyperlipidemia.* Am J Clin Nutr 1985; 45: 604–17.

5 Diabetes Nutrition Study Group of the European Association for the Study of Diabetes. *Nutritional recommendations for individuals with diabetes mellitus.* Diab Nutr Metab 1988; 1: 145–9.

6 American Diabetes Association. Position Statement. *Nutritional recommendations and principles for individuals with diabetes mellitus.* Diabetes Care 1990; 13 (suppl): 18–25.

7 Nutrition Subcommittee of the British Diabetic Association's Professional Advisory Committee. *Dietary recommendations for people with diabetes: an update for the 1990s.* J Hum Nutr Diet 1991; 4: 393–412.

8 Frost G, Wilding JPH. *Specific advice to use a low glycemic index diet improves metabolic control in newly diagnosed NIDDM.* Diabetic Medicine 1993; 10 (suppl): s29.

9 International Diabetes Institute. *Diabetes—eating for health.* Melbourne: International Diabetes Institute, 1994.

10 Shils ME, Olson JA, Shike M (eds). *Modern nutrition in health and disease.* Philadelphia: Lea and Febiger, 1994.

11 Collings P, Williams C, Macdonald I. *Effects of cooking on serum glucose and insulin responses.* BMJ; 282: 1032.

12 O'Dea K, Nestel PJ, Antonoff L. *Physical factors influencing post prandial glucose and insulin responses.* Am J Clin Nutr 1980; 33: 760–5.

13 Brand JC, Nicholson PL, Thorburn AW, Truswell AS. *Food processing and the glycemic index.* Am J Clin Nutr 1985; 42: 1192–6.

14 Heaton KW, Marcus SN, Emmett PM, Bolton CH. *Particle size of wheat, maize, and oat test meals: effects on plasma glucose and insulin responses and on the rate of starch digestion in vitro.* Am J Clin Nutr 1988; 47: 675–82.

15 Holt S, Brand Miller J. *Particle size, satiety and the glycemic response.* Eur J Clin Nutr 1994; 48: 496–502.

16 Ross SW, Brand JC, Thorburn AW, Truswell AS. *Glycemic index of processed wheat products.* Am J Clin Nutr 1987; 46: 631–5.

17 Granfeldt Y, Bjork I, Hagander B. *On the importance of processing conditions, product thickness and egg addition for the glycemic and hormonal responses to pasta: a comparison with bread made from "pasta ingredients."* Eur J Clin Nutr 1991; 45: 489–99.

18 Jenkins DJA, Wolever TMS, Jenkins AL, Lee R, Wong GS, Josse R. *Glycemic response to wheat products: reduced response to pasta but no effect of fibre.* Diabetes Care 1983; 6: 2: 155–9.

19 Brand Miller J, Pang E, Bramall L. *Rice: a high or low glycemic index food?* Am J Clin Nutr 1992; 56: 1034–6.

20 Thomas DE, Brotherhood JR, Brand JC. *Carbohydrate feeding before exercise: effect of glycemic index.* Internat J Sports Med 1991; 12: 180–6.

21 Holt S, Brand J, Soveny C, Hansky J. *Relationship of satiety to postprandial glycemic, insulin and cholecystokinin responses.* Appetite 1992; 18: 129–41.

22 Leathwood P, Pollet P. *Effects of slow release carbohydrates in the form of bean flakes on the evolution of hunger and satiety in man.* Appetite 1988; 10: 1–11.

23 Truswell AS. *Glycemic index of foods.* Eur J Clin Nutr 1992; 46: S91–S101.

24 Krezowski PA, Nuttall FQ, Gannon MC, Bartosh NH. *The effect of protein ingestion on the metabolic response to oral glucose in normal individuals.* Am J Clin Nutr 1986; 44: 847–56.

25 Wolever TMS, Katzman-Relle L, Jenkins AL, et al. *Glycemic index of 102 complex carbohydrate foods in patients with diabetes.* Nutr Res 1994; 14: 651–69.

26 Brand Miller JC, Broomhead L, Pang E. *Glycemic index of foods con-taining sugar.* Brit J Nutr 1995; 73, 613–23.

27 Krezowski PA, Nuttal FQ, Gannon MC, et al. *Insulin and glucose responses to various starch-containing foods in type II diabetic sub-jects.* Diabetes Care 1987; 10: 205–12.

28 Jenkins DJA, Wesson V, Wolever TMS, et al. *Wholemeal versus whole-grain breads: proportion of whole or cracked grain and the glycemic response.* BMJ 1988; 297: 958–60.

29 Granfeldt Y, Bjorck I, Drews A, Tovar J. *An in vitro procedure based on chewing to predict metabolic response to starch in cereal and legume products.* Eur J Clin Nutr 1992; 46: 649–60.

30 Brown D, Tomlinson D, Brand Miller J. *The development of low glycemic index breads.* Proc Nutr Soc Aust 1992; 17: 62.

31 Jenkins DJA, Wolever TMS, Jenkins AL, et al. *Low glycemic response to traditionally processed wheat and rye products: bulgur and pumper-nickel bread.* Am J Clin Nutr 1986; 43: 516–20.

32 Otto H, Niklas L. *Differences d'action sur la glycemie d'aliments con-tenant des hydrated de carbone: consequences pou le traitment diete-tique du diabete sucre.* Quoted in Jenkins DJA, Wolever TMS and Jenkins LA, *Starchy foods and glycemic index.* Diabetes Care 1988; 11: 149–59.

33 Wolever TMS, Jenkins DJA, Josse RG, Wong GS, Lee R. *The glycemic index: similarity of values derived in insulin-dependent and non-insulin-dependent diabetic patients.* J Am Coll Nut 1987; 6: 295–305.

34 Schauberger G, Brinck UC, Guldner G, Spaethe R, Niklas L, Otto H. *Exchange of carbohydrates according to their effect on blood glucose.* Quoted in Jenkins DJA, Wolever TMS, Jenkins AL, Josse RG, Wong GS. *The glycemic response to carbohydrate foods.* Lancet 1984; 1: 388–91.

35 Brand JC, Foster KA, Crossman S, Truswell AS. *The glycemic and insulin indices of realistic meals and rye breads tested in healthy sub-jects.* Diab Nutr Metab 1990; 3: 137–42.

36 Walker ARP, Walker BF. *Glycemic index of South African foods deter-mined in rural blacks—a population at low risk of diabetes.* Hum Nutr Clin Nutr 1984; 38C: 215–22.

37 Jenkins DJA, Wolever TMS, Jenkins AL, et al. *The glycemic index of foods tested in diabetic patients: A new basis for carbohydrate exchange favouring the use of legumes.* Diabetologia 1983; 24:

257–64.

38 Crapo PA, Kolterman OG, Waldeck N, Reaven GM, Olefsky JM. *Postprandial hormonal responses to different types of complex carbohydrate in individuals with impaired glucose tolerance.* Am J Clin Nutr 1980; 33: 1723–8.

39 Bornet FRJ, Costagliola D, Rizkalla SW, et al. *Insulinemic and glycemic indexes of six starch-rich foods taken alone and in a mixed meal by type 2 diabetics.* Am J Clin Nutr 1987; 45: 588–95.

40 Jenkins DJA, Thorne MJ, Wolever TMS, Jenkins AL, Rao AV, Thompson LU. *The effect of starch-protein interaction in wheat on the glycemic response and rate of in vitro digestion.* Am J Clin Nutr 1987; 45: 946–51.

41 Brand Miller JC, Bell, L, Denning K, Holt S. *In search of more low glycemic index foods.* Proc Nutr Soc Aust 1995; 19, 177.

42 Potter JG, Coffman KP, Reid RL, Drall JM, Albrink MJ. *Effect of test meals of varying dietary fibre content on plasma insulin and glucose response.* Am J Clin Nutr 1981; 34: 328–34.

43 Wolever TMS, Wong GS, Kenshole A, Josse RG, Thompson LU, Lam KY, Jenkins DJA. *Lactose in the diabetic diet: a comparison with other carbohydrates.* Nutr Res 1985; 5: 1335–45.

44 Crapo PA, Insel J, Sperling M, Kolterman OG. *Comparison of serum glucose, insulin and glucagon responses to different types of complex carbohydrate in non-insulin-dependent diabetic patients.* Am J Clin Nutr 1981; 34: 184–90.

45 Crapo PA, Reaven G, Olefsky J. *Postprandial plasma-glucose and - insulin responses to different complex carbohydrates.* Diabetes 1977; 26: 1178–83.

46 Wolever TMS, Nuttall FQ, Lee R, Wong GS, Josse RG, Csima A, Jenkins DJA. *Prediction of the relative blood glucose response of mixed meals using bread glycemic index.* Diabetes Care 1985; 8: 418–28.

47 Wolever TMS, Jenkins DJA, Kalmusky J et al. *Comparison of regular and parboiled rices: explanation of discrepancies between reported glycemic responses to rice.* Nutr Res 1986; 6: 349–57.

48 Rahman M, Malik MA, Mubarak SA. *Glycemic index of Pakistani staple foods in mixed meals for diabetics.* J Pak Med Assoc 1992; 42: 60–2.

49 Dilwari JB, Kamath PS, Batta RP, Mukewar S, Raghavan S. *Reduction of postprandial plasma glucose by bengal gram dal* (Cicer arietnum)

and rajmah (Phaseolus vulgaris*)*. Am J Clin Nutr 1981; 34: 2450–3.

50 Brand Miller JC, Holt S, Brammel L. Unpublished observation.

51 Kurup PG, Krishnamurthy S. *Glycemic index of selected foodstuffs commonly used in South India.* Internat J Vit Nutr Res 1992; 62: 266–8.

52 Rasmussen O, Gregersen S. *Influence of the amount of starch on the glycemic index to rice in non-insulin-dependent diabetic subjects.* Br J Nutr 1992; 67: 371–7.

53 Rasmussen OW, Gregersen S, Dørup J, Hermansen K. *Blood glucose and insulin responses to different meals in non-insulin-dependent diabetic subjects of both sexes.* Am J Clin Nutr 1992; 56: 712–5.

54 Buclossi A, Conti A, Lombardo S, Marsilii A, Petruzzi E, Piazza E, Pulini M. *Glycemic and inulinaemic responses to different carbohydrates in Type II (NIDD) diabetic patients.* Diab Nutr Metab 1990; 3: 143–51.

55 Gannon MC, Nuttall FQ, Krezowsky PA, Billington CJ, Parker S. *The serum insulin and plasma glucose responses to milk and fruit products in type 2 (non-insulin-dependent) diabetic patients.* Diabetologia 1986; 29: 784–91.

56 Bukar J, Mezitis NHE, Saitas V, Pi-Sunyer FX. *Frozen desserts and glycemic response in well-controlled NIDDM patients.* Diabetes Care 1990; 13: 4: 382–5.

57 Ha MA, Mann JI, Melton LD, Lewis-Barned NJ. *Relationship between the glycemic index and sugar content of fruits.* Diab Nutr Metab 1992; 5: 199–203.

58 Wolever TMS, Vuksan V, Katzman Relle L, Jenkins AL, Josse RG, Wong GS, Jenkins DJA. *Glycemic index of fruits and fruit products in patients with diabetes.* Int J Food Sc Nutr 1993; 43: 205–12.

59 Hermansen K, Rasmussen O, Gregersen S, Larsen S. *Influence of ripeness of banana on the blood glucose and insulin response in type 2 diabetic subjects.* Diabetic Medicine 1992; 9: 730–43.

60 Wolever TMS, Jenkins DJA, Thompson LU, et al. *Effect of canning on the blood glucose response to beans in patients with type 2 diabetes.* Hum Nutr Clin Nutr 1987; 41C: 135–40.

61 Vorster HH, van Tonder E, Kotzé JP, Walker ARP. *Effects of graded sucrose additions on taste preference, acceptability, glycemic index, and insulin response to butter beans.* Am J Clin Nutr 1987; 45: 575–9.

62 Jenkins DJA, Wolever TMS, Wong GS, Kenshole A, Josse RG,

Thompson LU, Lam KY. *Glycemic responses to foods: possible differences between insulin-dependent and non-insulin dependent diabetics.* Am J Clin Nutr 1984; 40: 971–81.

63 Fitz-Henry A. *In vitro and in vivo rates of carbohydrate digestion in Aboriginal bushfoods and contemporary Western foods.* Thesis submitted for BSc (Honours), Human Nutrition Unit, Department of Biochemistry, University of Sydney, October 1982.

64 Wolever TMS, Cohen Z, Thompson LU, Thorne MJ, Jenkins MJA, Prokipchuk EJ, Jenkins DJA. *Ileal loss of available carbohydrate in man: comparison of a breath hydrogen method with direct measurement using a human ileostomy model.* Am J Gastroenterol 1986; 81: 115–22.

65 Foster KA. *Glucose and insulin responses to legumes, pastas and rye breads.* Thesis submitted for BSc (Honours), Human Nutrition Unit, Department of Biochemistry, University of Sydney, October 1987.

66 Wolever TMS, Jenkins DJA, Kalmusky J, et al. *Glycemic response to pasta: effect of surface area, degree of cooking and protein enrichment.* Diabetes Care 1986; 9: 401–4.

67 Rasmussen O, Winther E, Arnfred J, Hermansen K. *Comparison of blood glucose and insulin responses in non-insulin dependent diabetic patients.* European J Clin Nutr 1988; 42: 953–61.

68 d'Emden MC, Marwick TH, Dreghorn J, Howlett VL, Cameron DP. *Postprandial glucose and insulin responses to different types of spaghetti and bread.* Diabetes Research and Clinical Practice 1987; 3: 221–6.

69 Wolever TMS, Kalmusky J, Giudici S, et al. *Effect of processing/preparation on the blood glucose response to potatoes.* Can Inst Food Sci Technol J 1985; 18(3): xxxv–xxxvi.

70 Frati-Munari AC, Roca-Vides RA, Lopez-Perez RJ, de Vivero I, Ruiz-Velazco M. *The glycemic index of some foods common in Mexico.* Gaac-Med-Mex 1991; 127: 163–70.

71 Brand JC, Snow BJ, Nabhan GP, Truswell AS. *Plasma glucose and insulin responses to traditional Pima Indian meals.* Am J Clin Nutr 1990; 51: 416–20.

72 Payne Y. *The glycemic index of six foods traditionally consumed by the Pima Indian tribe.* (Sydney University-Human Nutrition Unit) Master of Nutrition and Dietetics Research Essay, vol. 3, Section 12; 1992.

73 Mani UV, Prabhu SS, Damle SS, Mani I. *Glycemic index of some commonly consumed foods in Western India*. Asia Pacific J Clin Nutr 1993; 2: 111–4.

74 Shukla K, Narain JP, Puri P, Gupta A, Bijlani RL, Mahapatra SC, Karmarkar MG. *Glycemic response to maize, bajra and barley*. Indian J Physiol Pharmacol 1991; 35: 249–54.

75 Mani UV, Pradhan SN, Mehta NC, Thakur DM, Iyer U, Mani I. *Glycemic index of conventional carbohydrate meals*. Br J Nutr 1992; 68: 445–50.

76 Thorburn A. *Digestion and absorption of carbohydrate in Australian Aboriginal, Pacific Island and Western Foods*. Thesis submitted for Doctor of Philosophy, Human Nutrition Unit, Department of Biochemistry, University of Sydney, September 1986.

77 Lunetta M, DiMauro M, Crimi S, Mughini L. *No important differences in glycemic responses to common fruits in Type 2 diabetic patients*. Diab Med 1995; 12: 674–8.

78 Salmeron J, Manson JE, Stampfer MJ, Colditz GA, Wing AL, Willet WC. *Dietary fiber, glycemic load and risk of non-insulin-dependent diabetes mellitus in women*. JAMA 1997; 277: 472-77.

79 Salmeron J, Ascherio EB, Rimm GA, Colditz D, Spiegelman D, Jenkins DJ, Stampfer MJ, Wing AL, Willet WC. *Dietary fiber, glycemic load, and risk of NIDDM in men*. Diabetes Care 1997; 20: 545-50.

80 Liu S, Stampfer MJ, Manson JE, Hu FB, Franz M, Hennekens CH, Willet, WC. *A prospective study of dietary glycaemic load and risk of myocardial infarction in women*. FASEB 1998; 124: A260 (abstract #1517).

81 Frost G, Keogh B, Smith D, Akinsanya K, Leeds AR. *The effect of low glycaemic carbohydrate on insulin and glucose response in vivo and in vitro in patients with coronary heart disease*. Metabolism 1995; 45: 669-72.

82 Frost G, Keogh B, Smith DK, Leeds AR. *Differences in glucose uptake in adipocutes from patients with and without coronary heart disease*. Diabetic Medicine 1998; 15: 1003-9.

83 Frost G, Trew G, Margara R, Leeds AR, Dornhorst A. *Improvement in adipocyte insulin response to a low glycaemic index diet in women at risk of cardiovascular disease*. Metabolism 1998; 47(10): 1245-51.

84 Frost G, Leeds AR, Dore CJB, Madieros S, Brading S, Dornhorst A.

Glycaemic index as a determinant of serum high density lipoprotein. Lancet 1999; 353: 1045-8.
85 Soh NL, Brand-Miller, J. *The glycemic index of potatoes: effect of variety, cooking method and maturity.* Eur J Clin Nutr 1998; 52: 1-6.

ACKNOWLEDGMENTS

The first edition of this book was published in Australia in 1996 under the title *The G.I. Factor*. In 1998, a completely revised edition was published, and that same year the book was also published in the United Kingdom.

This new edition, *The Glucose Revolution*, has been revised and completely adapted for the North American market. We gratefully acknowledge the essential role of adapter Johanna Burani, M.S., R.D., C.D.E., who has worked tirelessly to make the book accurate and appropriate for North American readers.

Many people have contributed to this book and we sincerely thank them all. Special thanks go to our meticulous editors, Matthew Lore at Marlowe & Company, and Philippa Sandall at Hodder Australia, who put their faith in us and brought the book to fruition. Many nutrition students and volunteers from the Human Nutrition Unit of the University of Sydney undertook glycemic index testing. Susanne Holt and Diana Thomas masterminded the satiety and athletic performance studies and Kellogg Australia generously funded their research. Isa Hopwood typed up the original glycemic index table. Dietitians Catherine Saxelby, Shirley Crossman, Rudi Bartl, Helen O'Connor, and Martina Chippendall contributed to various chapters. Thanks to Rick Mendosa for his indefatigable support of this book on the Internet and his thorough review of the U.S. edition. Lastly, we thank our long-suffering spouses for their humor and unswerving (well, most of the time) support.

INDEX

RECIPE INDEX

GLYCEMIC INDEX TESTING

If you are a food manufacturer, you may be interested in having the glycemic index of some of your products tested on a fee-for-service basis. (A summary of the glycemic index testing procedure appears on page 26.) For more information, contact either:

Glycaemic Index Testing Inc.
135 Mavety Street
Toronto, Ontario
Canada M6P 2L8
E-mail: thomas.wolever@utoronto.ca

or

Sydney University Glycaemic Index Research Service (SUGIRS)
Department of Biochemistry
University of Sydney
NSW 2006 Australia
Fax: (61) (2) 9351-6022
E-mail: j.brandmiller@staff.usyd.edu.au

ABOUT THE AUTHORS

Jennie Brand-Miller, Ph.D., Associate Professor of Human Nutrition in the Human Nutrition Unit, Department of Biochemistry, University of Sydney, Australia, is widely recognized as one of the world's leading authorities on the glycemic index. She received her B.Sc. (1975) and Ph.D. (1979) degrees from the Department of Food Science and Technology at the University of New South Wales, Australia. She is the Editor of the *Proceedings of the Nutrition Society of Australia* and a member of the Scientific Consultative Committee of the Australian Nutrition Foundation. She has written more than 200 research papers, including 60 on the glycemic index of foods. She lives in Sydney, Australia.

Thomas M.S. Wolever, M.D., Ph.D., another of the world's leading researchers of the glycemic index, is Professor in the Department of Nutritional Sciences, University of Toronto, and a member of the Division of Endocrinology and Metabolism, St. Michael's Hospital, Toronto. He is a graduate of Oxford University (B.A., M.A., M.B., B.Ch., M.Sc., and D.M.) in the United Kingdom. He received his Ph.D. at the University of Toronto. His research since 1980 has focused on the glycemic index of foods and the prevention of type 2 diabetes. He lives in Toronto, Canada.

Stephen Colagiuri, M.D., is President of the Australian Diabetes Society, director of the Diabetes Center, and head of the Department of Endocrinology, Metabolism, and Diabetes at the Prince of Wales Hospital, Randwick, New South Wales, Australia. He is a graduate of the University of Sydney (MBBS, 1970) and a member of the Royal Australasian College of Physicians (1977). He has joint academic appointments at the University of New South Wales. He has authored more than 100 scientific papers, many concerned with the importance of carbohydrate in the diet of people with diabetes. He lives in Sydney, Australia.

Kaye Foster-Powell, B.Sc., M.Nutr. & Diet., is an accredited dietitian-nutritionist in both public and private practice in New South Wales, Australia. A graduate of the University of Sydney (B.Sc., 1987; Masters of Nutrition and Dietetics, 1994), she has extensive experience in diabetes management and has researched practical applications of the glycemic index over the last five years. She lives in Sydney, Australia.

Johanna Burani, M.S., R.D., C.D.E., is a registered dietitian and certified diabetes educator with more than 10 years experience in nutritional counseling. The author of seven books and professional manuals, she specializes in designing individual meal plans based on low glycemic index food choices. She lives in Mendham, New Jersey.